An Introduction to Mushroom

Edited by Ajit Kumar Passari and Sergio Sánchez

Published in London, United Kingdom

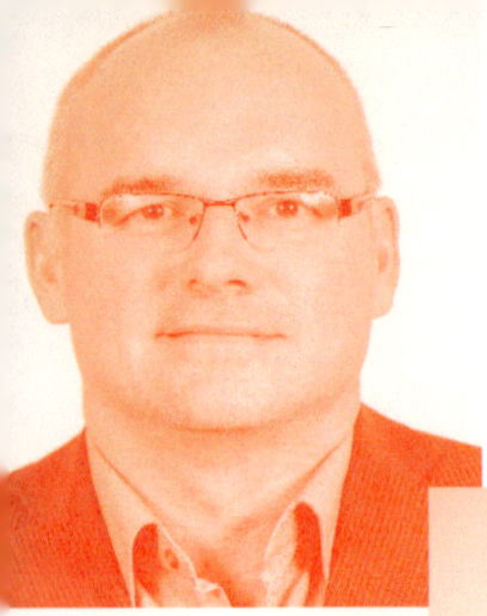
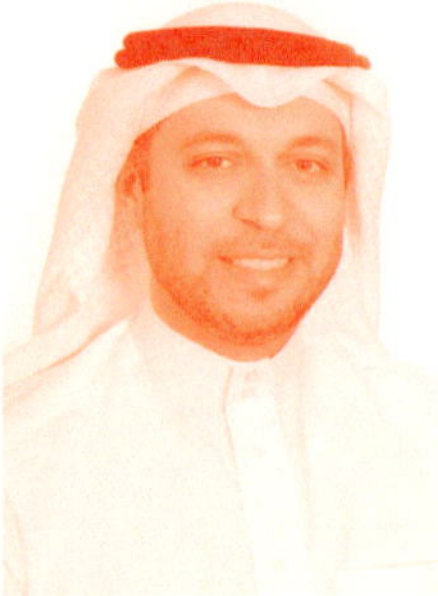
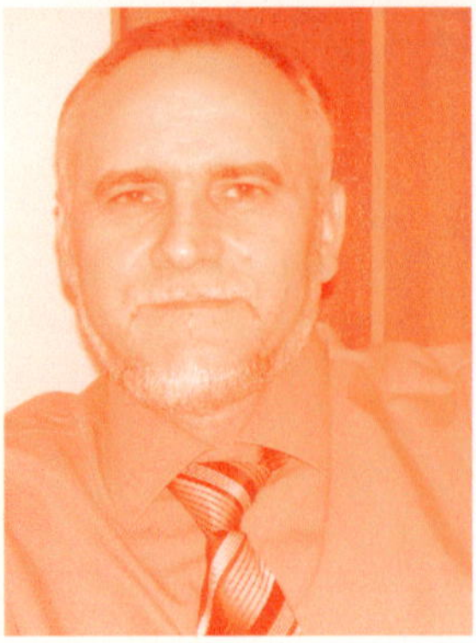
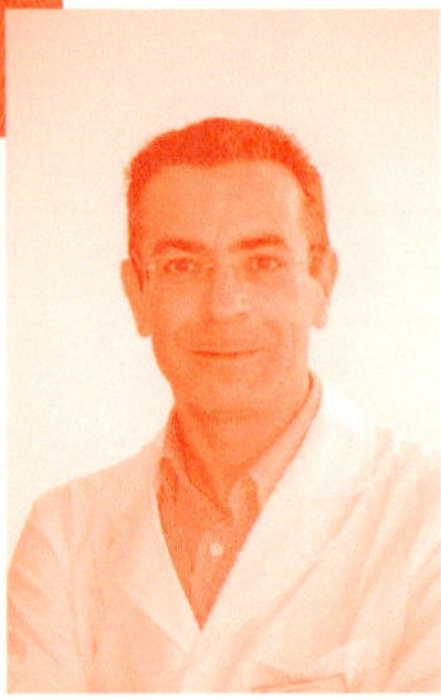
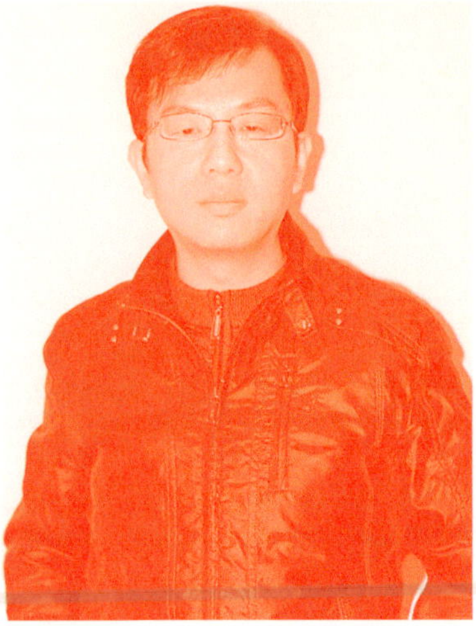
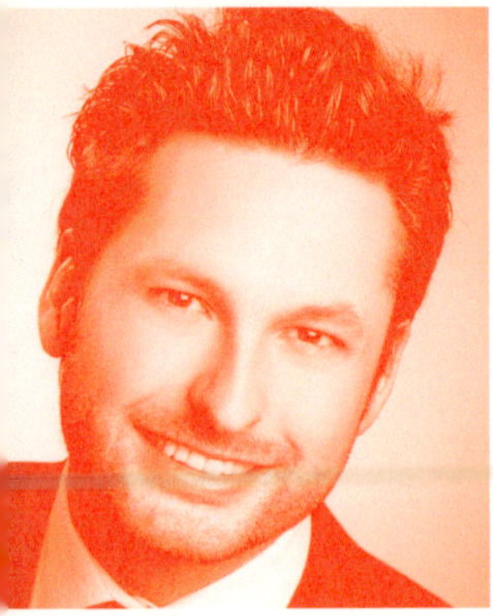
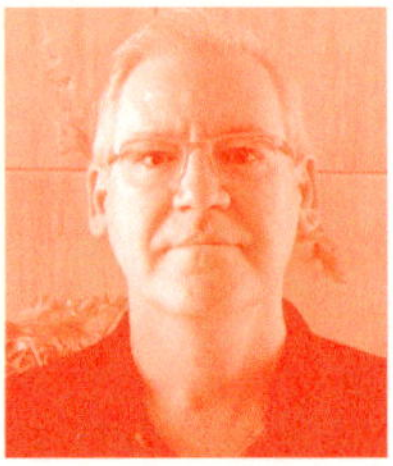

IntechOpen

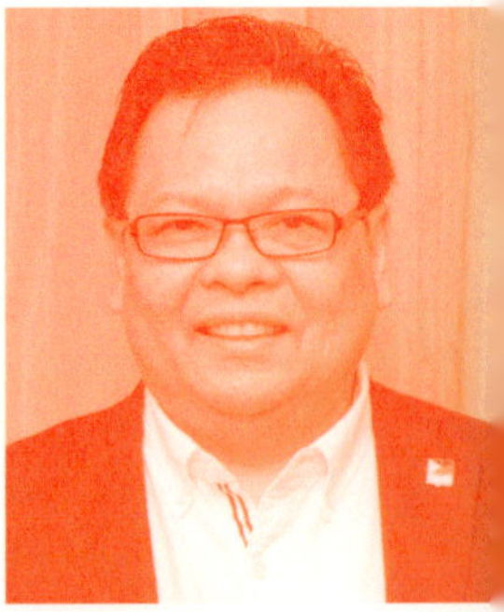
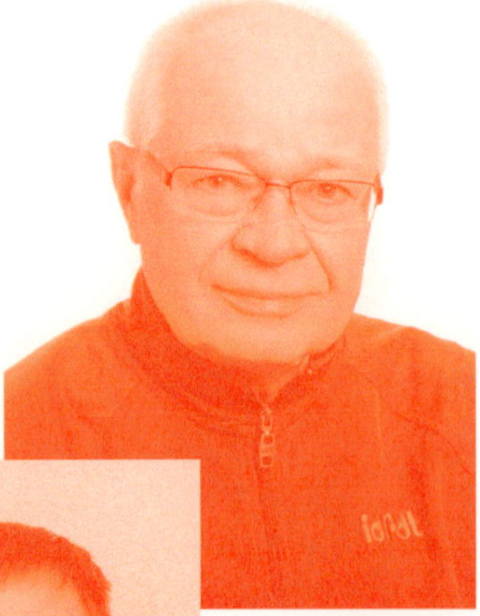
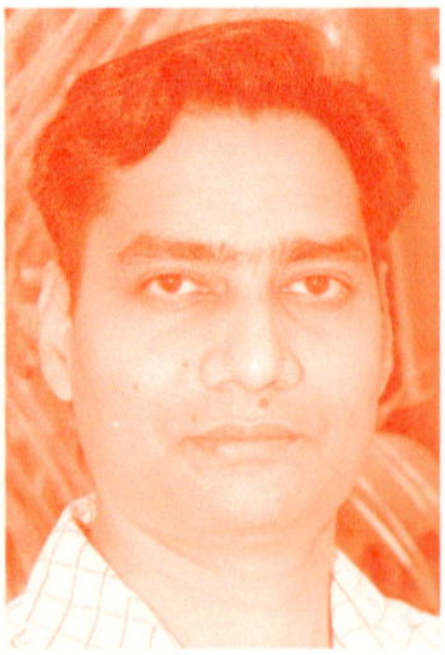
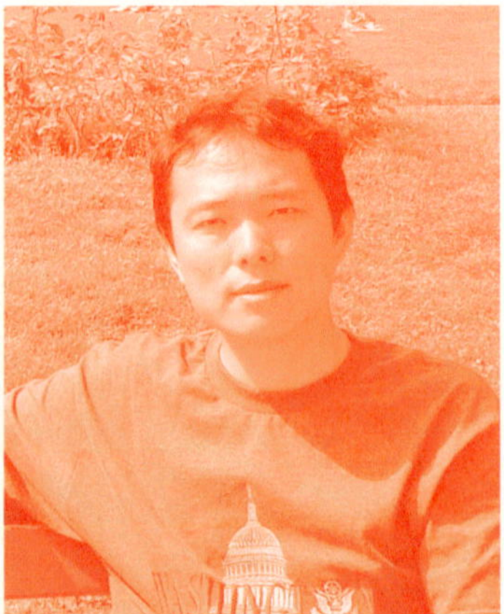
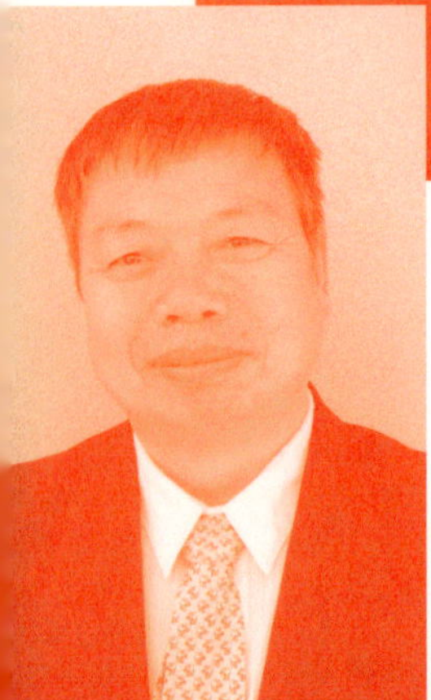
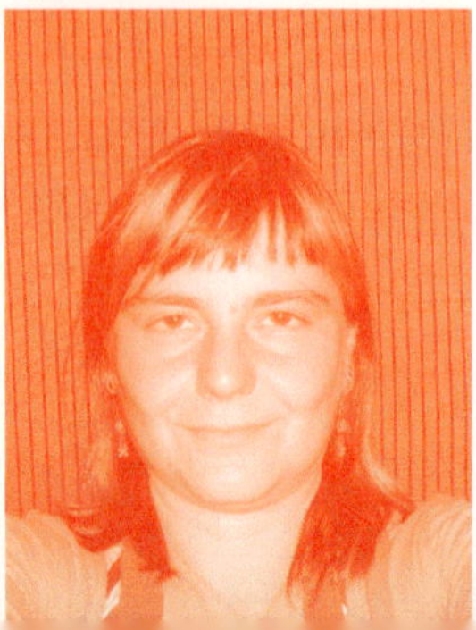

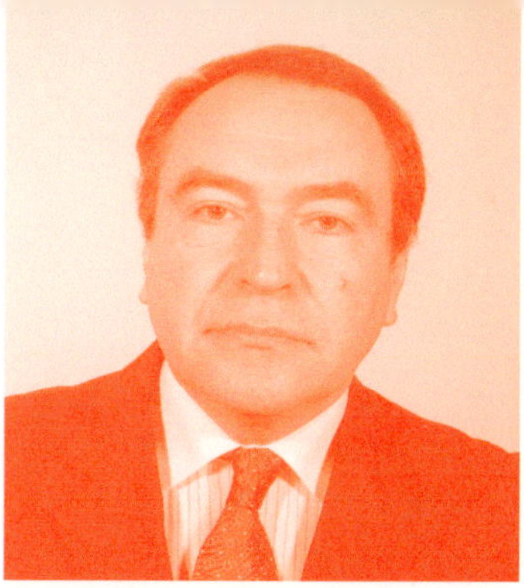
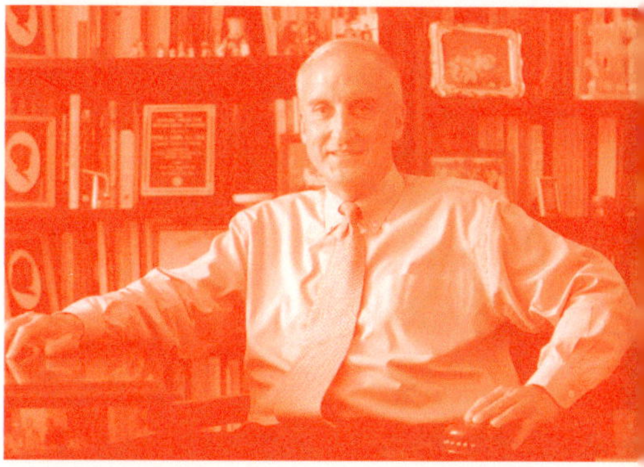
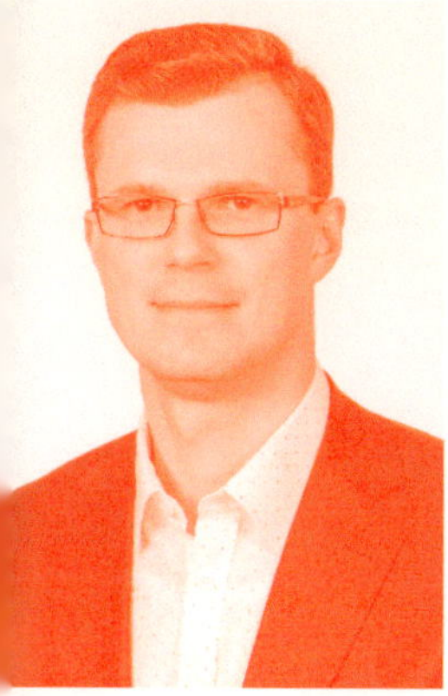
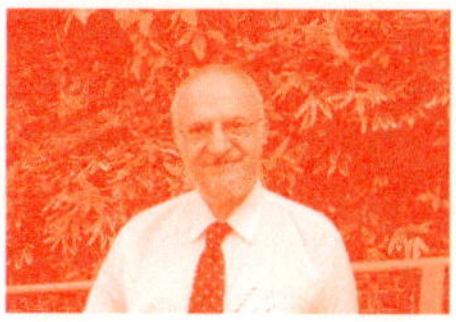
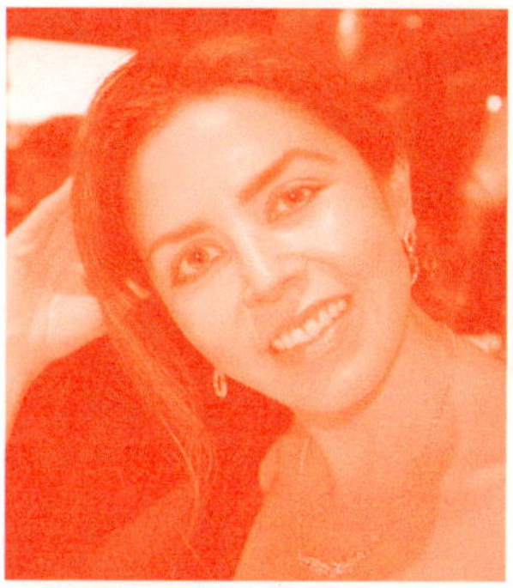

Supporting open minds since 2005

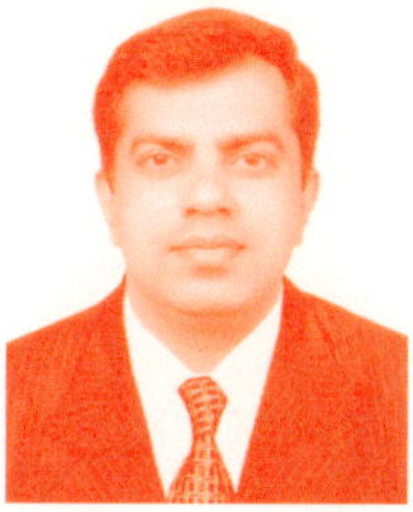
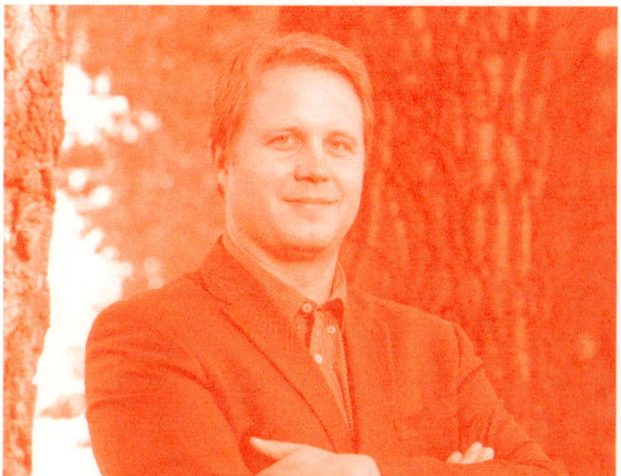
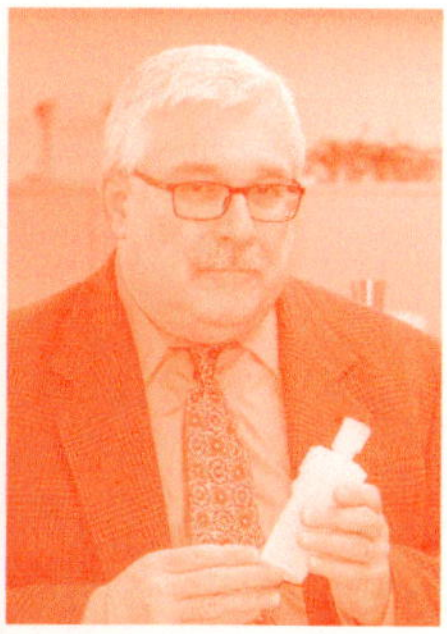
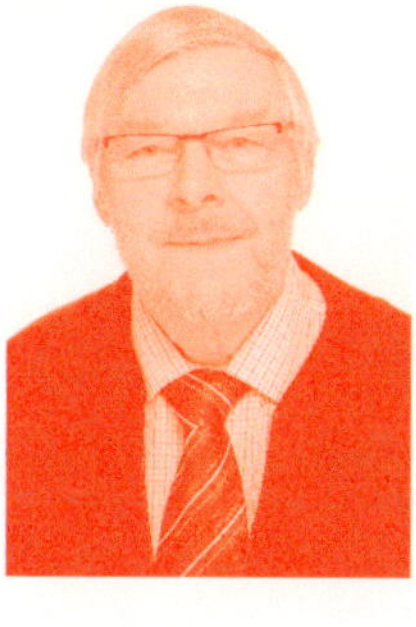
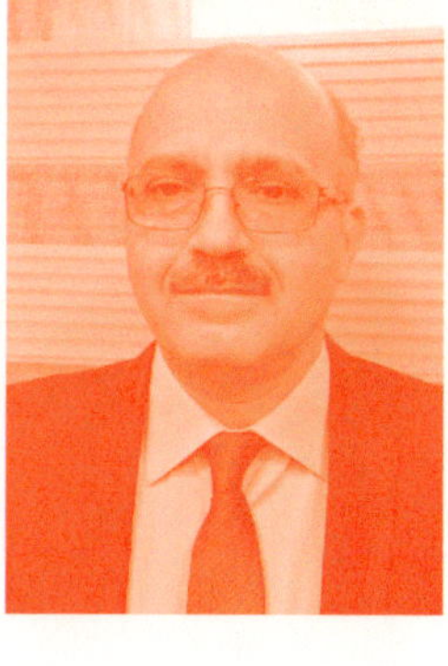
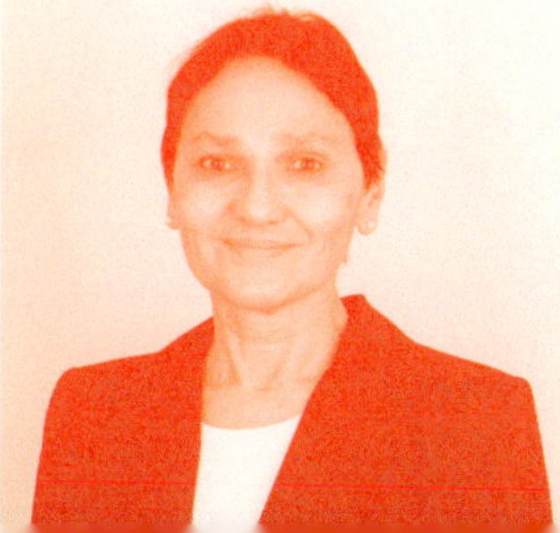
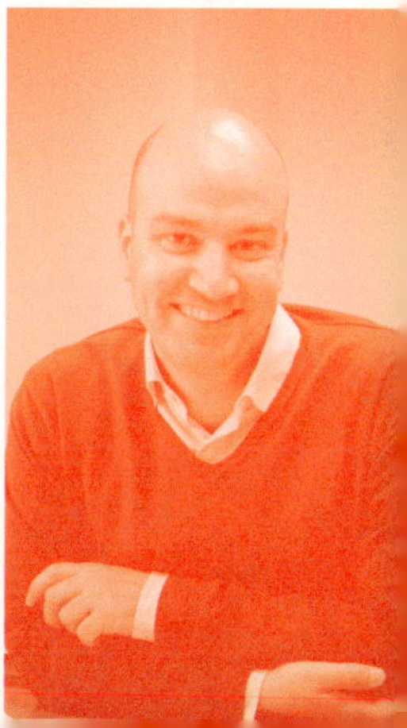

An Introduction to Mushroom
http://dx.doi.org/10.5772/intechopen.86908
Edited by Ajit Kumar Passari and Sergio Sánchez

Contributors
Moyen Uddin, Rumana Pervin, Rabiul Islam, Sourav Ahmed, Matiar Rahman, Sunita Bandopadhyay Mukhopadhyay, Gabriela Balogh, Diego Aguilera Braico, Ajit Kumar Passari, Maria Paula Gómez Román, Nathalia Badillo Mantilla, Sergio Andrés Carreño Flórez, Rodríguez Sanoja Romina, Beatriz Ruiz Villafan, Sergio Sánchez, Surajit De Mandal, Udaya Kumar Vandana, Pranab Behari Mazumder, Abu Barkat Md Gulzar, Lee Hoon Ho, Noroul Asyikeen Zulkifli, Thuan-Chew Tan, Clement Olusola Ogidi, Victor Olusegun Oyetayo, Bamidele Juliet Akinyele, Jabin Jahan, Prosenjit Paul

First published in London, United Kingdom, 2020 by IntechOpen
IntechOpen is the global imprint of INTECHOPEN LIMITED, registered in England and Wales, registration number: 11086078, 7th floor, 10 Lower Thames Street, London, EC3R 6AF, United Kingdom
Printed in Croatia

British Library Cataloguing-in-Publication Data
A catalogue record for this book is available from the British Library

Additional hard and PDF copies can be obtained from orders@intechopen.com

An Introduction to Mushroom
Edited by Ajit Kumar Passari and Sergio Sánchez
p. cm.
Print ISBN 978-1-78985-955-3
Online ISBN 978-1-78985-956-0
eBook (PDF) ISBN 978-1-83881-046-7

For EU product safety concerns:
IN TECH d.o.o., Prolaz Marije Krucifikse Kozulić 3, 51000 Rijeka, Croatia, info@intechopen.com or visit our website at intechopen.com.

Meet the editors

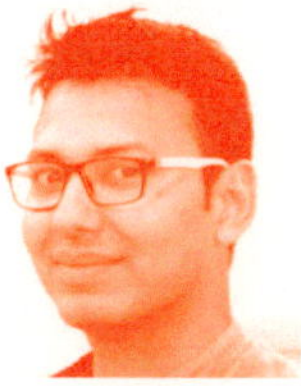

Dr Ajit Kumar Passari is working as a Postdoctoral Scientist in the Instituto de Investigaciones Biomédicas, Universidad Nacional Autónoma de México. Dr Passari has more than eight years of research experience in the fields of molecular biology, secondary metabolites production, PGPR, genomics, and metabolomics. Dr Passari has received multiple awards like *SNI Nacional Investigador Level I* under Conacyt funding of Gobierno De Mexico (2019) and *Young Scientist Award* at Nanyang Technological University, Singapore (2017).

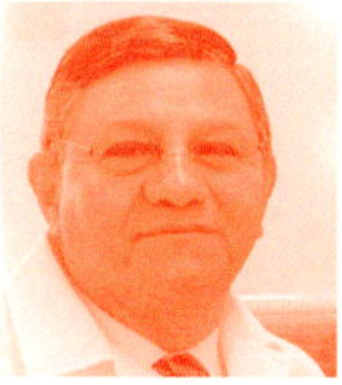

Prof. Sergio Sánchez is working as Professor in the Instituto de Investigaciones Biomédicas, Universidad Nacional Autónoma de México, and has more than fifty years of research experience in the fields of genomics, molecular biology, proteomics, secondary metabolites production, transcriptomics, and PGPR. Prof. Sánchez has been awarded several honors like Fellow, National Institutes of Health in 1974-1975, and Fellow, Consejo Nacional de Ciencia y Tecnología in 1973-1974.

Contents

Preface **XI**

Chapter 1 **1**
Antimicrobial and Antioxidant Potential of Wild Edible Mushrooms
by Maria Paula Gómez Román, Nathalia Badillo Mantilla, Sergio Andrés Carreño Flórez, Surajit De Mandal, Ajit Kumar Passari, Beatriz Ruiz-Villáfan, Romina Rodríguez-Sanoja and Sergio Sánchez

Chapter 2 **19**
Edible Mushroom: Nutritional Properties, Potential Nutraceutical Values, and Its Utilisation in Food Product Development
by Lee-Hoon Ho, Noroul Asyikeen Zulkifli and Thuan-Chew Tan

Chapter 3 **39**
Oyster Mushroom Cultivation on Water Hyacinth Biomass: Assessment of Yield Performances, Nutrient, and Toxic Element Contents of Mushrooms
by Sunita Bandopadhyay Mukhopadhyay

Chapter 4 **53**
Mushroom Polysaccharides: Chemistry and Anticancer Potentials
by Moyen Uddin Pk, Rumana Pervin, Jabin Jahan, Rabiul Islam Talukder, Sourav Ahmed and Matiar Rahman

Chapter 5 **65**
Molecular Mechanism Induced by Beta-Glucans from Maitake to Recover T Cell-Subpopulations during Immunosuppression
by Aguilera Braico Diego Maximo and Balogh Gabriela Andrea

Chapter 6 **93**
The Role of Mushrooms in Biodegradation and Decolorization of Dyes
by Abu Barkat Md Gulzar, Udaya Kumar Vandana, Prosenjit Paul and Pranab B. Mazumder

Chapter 7 **115**
Wild Medicinal Mushrooms: Potential Applications in Phytomedicine and Functional Foods
by Clement Olusola Ogidi, Victor Olusegun Oyetayo and Bamidele Juliet Akinyele

Preface

Mushrooms have often been referred to as a functional food due to their high nutritional content. They have many medicinal properties such as being an antioxidant, antimicrobial, anticancer, antidiabetic, immune enhancer, and also used for the treatment of various diseases such as anthelmintic, anti-inflammatory, antipyretics, etc. According to current information, there are approximately twelve-thousand species in the world, and out of them, 2000 species are reported as being edible. Around 35 edible mushroom varieties are cultivated commercially, whereas almost 200 wild species could be used for medicinal purposes. Mushrooms produce various types of extracellular enzymes that are useful for industry and also have the ability to decolorize dyes, which are very harmful to the environment. The present volume consists of seven chapters written by researchers from different countries, including the USA, Nigeria, Kenya, Brazil, Bangladesh, and India. This book covers most of the recent information about edible mushrooms and their applications as an alternative source for food production and biomedical fields. The editors express their robust appreciation to all the contributors for sharing their knowledge and ideas in this volume. The editors are also thankful to IntechOpen publishers for giving us a chance to amass this critical volume. We hope that the chapters presented in this book will be beneficial for students and researchers engaged in the mushroom research area.

Ajit Kumar Passari and Sergio Sánchez
National Autonomous University of Mexico,
Mexico

Chapter 1

Antimicrobial and Antioxidant Potential of Wild Edible Mushrooms

Maria Paula Gómez Román, Nathalia Badillo Mantilla, Sergio Andrés Carreño Flórez, Surajit De Mandal, Ajit Kumar Passari, Beatriz Ruiz-Villáfan, Romina Rodríguez-Sanoja and Sergio Sánchez

Abstract

Wild edible mushrooms have a high nutritional property that has been consumed by people from different parts of the world, producing a wide variety of bioactive compounds such as polysaccharides, peptides, glycoproteins, triterpenoids, lipids, and their derivatives. In the world, multidrug-resistant pathogens have been increasing drastically, and it is very urgent to search for alternative solutions to fight against multidrug-resistant pathogens. Moreover, unhealthy foods, ultraviolet radiation, as well as other environmental effects, are responsible for generating free radicals, oxidative stress, and numerous health diseases. Hence, the wild edible mushroom could be an alternative source of new antimicrobial potential and possesses antioxidant properties that can play significant roles in preventing various health diseases. In this book chapter, we focus on investigating the antimicrobial and antioxidant potential of wild edible mushrooms and their bioactive compound production.

Keywords: edible mushrooms, antimicrobial, antioxidant, bioactive compounds

1. Introduction

Fungi are eukaryotic and spore-bearing organisms with a life cycle divided into two phases: a growth phase and a reproductive phase. Macro fungi or mushrooms are species with a natural fruit body that can grow large enough to be visible or can grow underground. The spores, produced by the fruiting body, are the unit of sexual and asexual reproduction and are responsible for fungi's spread [1].

About 14,000 mushroom species have been reported, among them, 2000 mushrooms are reported as edible [2]. Additionally, less than 1% of the recognized fungus is poisonous, and a less percentage is fatal species [3]. Edible mushrooms have high medicinal properties due to their great rich content of polysaccharides, especially β-glucans. Many researchers reported that edible mushrooms have enormous features, including antioxidants, cholesterol-lowering properties, anti-hypertensive, anti-inflammatory, liver protection, as well as anti-diabetic, anti-viral, and anti-microbial potential (**Figure 1**) [4–7].

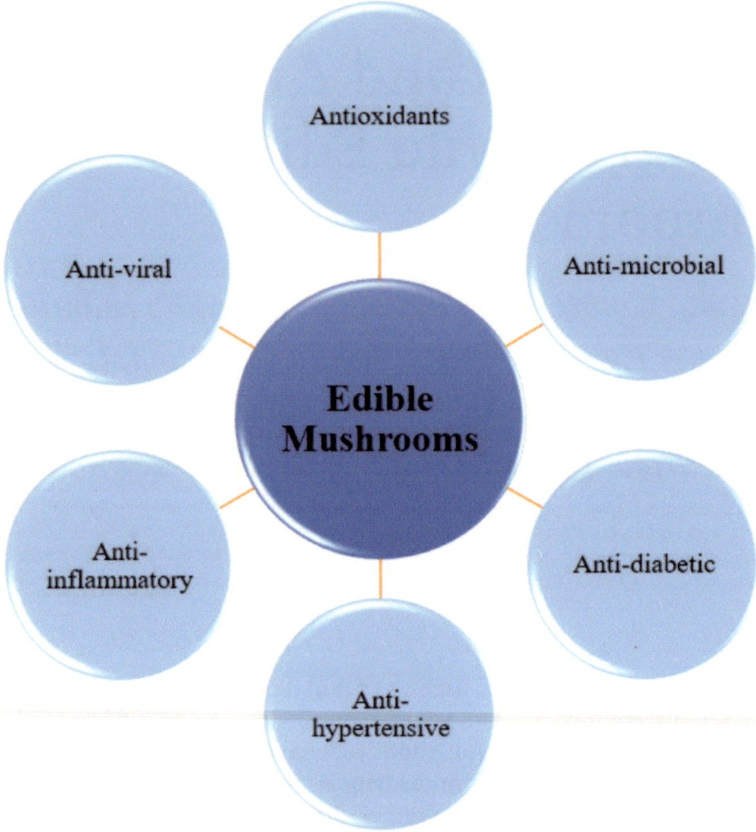

Figure 1.
Properties of edible mushrooms.

Currently, antimicrobial drug resistance is the serious problem in the world. The selection of bacterial strains based on physiological or biological aspects used high doses for the treatment of antimicrobial resistance pathogens [8]. Under certain conditions, the susceptible bacterial growth is inhibited by the drug while it becomes high resistant [9]. This problem has eagerly vigored the researchers to find the alternative source to fight against multidrug resistant pathogens and develop the new antimicrobial substances from various sources [10]. Hence, the researchers are studied that various types of mushroom have high antimicrobial potential and could be useful for new therapeutic activities such as anticarcinogenic, immuno-suppressor, and antibiotic, among others. In recent periods, different genus mushroom (*Lycoperdon* sp., *Cantharellus* sp., *Agaricus* sp., *Clavaria* sp., and *Pleurotus* sp.) extracts showing great interest as an alternative source to obtain natural products from the various researchers [11]. Various solvents like methanol, acetone and hexane was used to prepare mushroom extracts that showed significant antimicrobial activities [12, 13]. Edible mushrooms have been used in health care for treating diseases for their compelling bioactive compound content. The most widely cultivated mushrooms are *Agaricus bisporus*, *Lentinus edodes*, *Pleurotus* spp., and *Flammulina velutipes* [14], which showed the most considerable antimicrobial activity against Gram-positive and Gram-negative bacteria. Thus, it is essential to be a focus on studying different types of edible mushroom extracts to find a source of physiologically beneficial and non-toxic medicines against the multidrug-resistant pathogens [12].

Moreover, full edible mushrooms show significant antioxidant activity. Antioxidant compounds protect the cells from oxidative stress, a cellular process involved in the development of different humans' diseases as diabetic disease, Alzheimer's disease, and cancer, among others. Hence, it is necessary to investigate the different extracts of mushroom displayed potent antioxidant activity. For example, *Melanoleuca* species could be considered for pharmacological studies because of its high antioxidant capacity [15]. Additionally, a few researchers suggested that higher content of antioxidants present in the mushroom could be used as a food supplement that can supply high nutrient ability in the body [16, 17].

As we know, edible mushrooms have wide range of industrial and pharmaceutical applications. In this chapter, we will focus to describe the importance of wild edible mushrooms with their antimicrobial potential against pathogens as well as determine their antioxidant activities.

2. General information about mushroom

Mushrooms are eukaryotic heterotrophic organisms defined as macrofungi with a fruiting body formed by a cap and a stalk [18]. These macrofungi contain a wide variety of species belonging to the class Basidiomycota [19]. The mushrooms are filamentous fungi with both sexual and asexual reproduction cycle. The characteristic of basidiomycetes is a spore-producing structure or fruiting body called basidium. The morphological unit of the basidium is the hyphae, and a mass of hyphae is called mycelium. The spores produced inside the basidium are called basidiospore and are responsible for its reproduction and its dissemination. Sexual reproduction begins when the basidiospore germinates and grown as a haploid mycelium in optimal environmental conditions [1, 20]. Mushrooms are well-known as edible and non-edible macro-fungi. The edible and non-edible mushroom can differentiate based on morphological characteristics like color, appearance, and shape of the cap [3].

In recent years, many studies have been reported that mushroom has extreme nutritional properties like vitamins, fats, proteins, etc. and could have high therapeutic properties that can be used as an antioxidant, anticancer, antidiabetic, cardiovascular protector, and hepatoprotective effects [19]. Moreover, the mushroom could be used as potential sources to obtain peptides, vitamins, proteins, lipids, amino acids, fiber, and antimicrobial compounds [14]. Last 20 years, most of the food industry could use the mushroom as a food product to prepare different kinds of jam, pickle, sweets, etc. [21].

3. Antimicrobial potential of edible mushroom

The use of antibiotics is the single most crucial factor leading to increased resistance of pathogenic microorganisms around the world [22]. Antibiotics are among the most commonly prescribed drugs used in human medicine. However, up to 50% of all the antibiotics prescribed for people are not needed or not optimally effective as prescribed [23]. Another major factor in the growth of antibiotic resistance is spread of the resistant strains of bacteria from person to person, or from the non-human sources in the environment, including food [24]. Natural resources have been taken advantage over the years, and among them, wild edible mushrooms vast diversity of active compounds with nutritional and antimicrobials properties [25–27]. Mushrooms have long been playing an essential role in several aspects, having medicinal value; mushrooms have been playing an indispensable role in several aspects of human activity, like feed and medicinal properties [28, 29]. Current researches have been focused on searching for new antimicrobials therapeutically potential compounds of edible mushrooms [22] recognizing that some of these molecules have health beneficial effects, including antimicrobial properties.

Mushroom	Extracts	Activity against	Method	References
Boletus lupinus; Flammulina velutipes, Phellinus igniarius, Sarcodon imbricatus, Tricholoma aurantium, Xerocomus ichnussanus	Methanol	*Escherichia coli, Staphylococcus aureus, Pseudomonas aeruginosa, Bacillus pumilus, Sarcina lutea*, and *Bacillus subtilis*	MIC = 2.5–50 mg/mL	Nikolovska et al. [33]
Pleurotus eryngii	Sulphated polysaccharides and crude polysaccharides	*Staphylococcus aureus, Listeria monocytogenes*, and *Escherichia coli*	MIC = 0.625–10.0 mg/mL and IZ = 11.7–31.8 mm	Li and Shah [34]
Coriolus versicolor	Methanol	*Staphylococcus epidermidis, Staphylococcus aureus, Bacillus cereus, Listeria monocytogenes, Shigella sonnei, Yersinia enterocolitica, Salmonella ser.* Enteritidis, and *Proteus hauseri*	MIC = 0.625–20.0 mg/mL and MBC = 1.25–40.0 mg/mL	Matijasevic et al. [35]
Lactarius deliciosus	Methanol	*Staphylococcus aureus, Bacillus subtilis, Bacillus cereus, Escherichia coli*, and *Proteus mirabilis*	MIC = 2.5–20.0 mg/mL	Kosanić et al. [36]
Macrolepiota procera	Methanol	*Staphylococcus aureus, Bacillus subtilis, Bacillus cereus, Escherichia coli*, and *Proteus mirabilis*	MIC = 5.0–10.0 mg/mL	Kosanić et al. [36]
Agaricus bisporus, Pleurotus ostreatus, and *Lentinula edodes*	Methanol	*Enterococcus faecalis, Methicillin sensitive Staphylococcus aureus, Methicillin resistant Staphylococcus aureus, Escherichia coli*, and *Pseudomonas aeruginosa*	MIC = 0.1–0.2 mg/mL	Taofiq et al. [37]
Verpa bohemica	Butanol and ethyl acetate	*Staphylococcus aureus, Escherichia coli*, and *Pseudomonas aeruginosa*	MIC = 250–750 μg/mL and MBC = 500–750 μg/mL	Shameem et al. [38]
Agaricus lanipes	Methanol	*Micrococcus luteus, Staphylococcus aureus, Bacillus subtilis, Proteus vulgaris, Escherichia coli*, and *Yersinia enterocolitica*	IZ = 11 ± 0–22 ± 1 mm	Kaygusuz et al. [39]
Lignosus rhinocerotis	Petroleum, chloroform, methanol and aqueous	*Staphylococcus, Streptococcus, Micrococcus, Corynebacterium, Bacillus, Klebsiella, Serratia, Salmonella, Pseudomonas*, and *Escherichia*	IZ = 7.0–17.67 mm	Mohanarji et al. [40]; Nallathamby et al. [41]

DOI: http://dx.doi.org/10.5772/intechopen.90945

Mushroom	Extracts	Activity against	Method	References
Flammulina velutipes	Ethyl-acetate	*Bacillus cereus, Enterobacter aerogenes, Escherichia coli, Micrococcus luteus, Proteus vulgaris, Salmonella typhimurium*, and *Staphylococcus aureus*	IZ = 7.0 ± 0.10–10.0 ± 0.50 mm and MIC = 2.50 ± 0.5–22.5 ± 1.7 mg/mL	Chaiharn et al. [32]
Ganoderma lucidum	Ethyl-acetate, methanol, aqueous, and ethanol	*Bacillus cereus, Enterobacter aerogenes, Escherichia coli, Micrococcus luteus, Proteus vulgaris, Salmonella typhimurium*, and *Staphylococcus aureus*	IZ = 6.2–20.0 mm and MIC = 1.50–25.0 mg/mL	Chaiharn et al. [32]
Pleurotus ostreatus	Ethyl-acetate, methanol, and ethanol	*Bacillus cereus, Enterobacter aerogenes, Escherichia coli, Micrococcus luteus, Proteus vulgaris, Salmonella typhimurium*, and *Staphylococcus aureus*	IZ = 6.1–12.0 mm and MIC = 1.50–17.5 mg/mL	Chaiharn et al. [32]
Pleurotus pulmonarius	Ethyl-acetate and aqueous	*Bacillus cereus, Enterobacter aerogenes, Escherichia coli, Micrococcus luteus, Proteus vulgaris, Salmonella typhimurium*, and *Staphylococcus aureus*	IZ = 6.1–15.0 mm and MIC = 1.25–15.5 mg/mL	Chaiharn et al. [32]
Leucoagaricus leucothites	Ethanol	*Pseudomonas aeruginosa, Escherichia coli, Enterococcus faecalis*, and *Staphylococcus aureus.*	MIC = 100–400 μg/mL	Sevindik et al. [42]
Craterellus cornucopioides	Acetone	*Bacillus cereus, Bacillus subtilis, Escherichia coli, Proteus mirabilis*, and *Staphylococcus aureus*	MIC = 0.1–0.2 mg/mL	Kosanić et al. [30]
Tricholoma equestre	Aqueous, methanol, cyclohexane, and dichloromethane	*Staphylococcus aureus, Bacillus subtilis, Enterococcus faecalis, Escherichia coli, Klebsiella pneumoniae, Salmonella abony*, and *Pseudomonas aeruginosa*	MIC = 250–500 μg/mL	Muszyńska et al. [43]

MIC-minimum bactericidal concentration; MBC-minimum inhibitory concentration; IZ-inhibition zone (disc diffusion).

Table 1.
Mushroom extracts with antimicrobial activity against Gram-positive and Gram-negative bacteria.

Nowadays, researchers are interested in searching antimicrobial compounds isolated from edible mushrooms that can be useful to inhibit the multidrug-resistant (MDR) pathogens. Recently, Kosanić et al. [30] state that acetone extract of Craterellus cornucopioides has strong minimum inhibitory concentration (MIC) against Gram-positive (Staphylococcus aureus, Bacillus cereus, and Bacillus subtilis) and Gram negative (Escherichia coli and Proteus mirabilis) bacteria with a range of 0.1–0.2 mg/mL. Interestingly, the effect of feeding C57BL/6 mice *Agaricus bisporous* (white button mushroom) was used to feed in mice and to evaluate the bacterial microflora, urinary metabolome, and resistance to a gastrointestinal (GI) pathogen along with control untreated mushroom. As a result, mice treat with mushrooms increased the diversity of the microflora and decreased the GI tract *Clostridia* pathogen [31]. Chaiharn et al. [32] reported that different types of extracts such as ethyl-acetate, methanol, and ethanol and aqueous solvent of *Flammulina velutipes, Ganoderma lucidum*, *Pleurotus ostreatus*, and *Pleurotus pulmonarius* showed significant antibacterial activity against Gram-positive and Gram-negative bacterial pathogens (**Table 1**).

4. Antioxidant potential of edible mushroom

Free radical is unstable and very reactive molecules defined as any molecule containing unpaired electrons. These molecules attack nearby chemical compounds to capture the needed electron for gaining stability [44, 45]. Free radicals can be derivate from nitrogen compounds [Reactive Nitrogen Species (RNS)] or molecular oxygen (O_2) [Reactive Oxygen Species (ROS)]. ROS are the ruling class of radical species producing by endogenous and exogenous sources in living systems [25]. The endogenous source is present in aerobic cells that include metabolism of energy production, respiratory burst, respiratory chain inside the mitochondrial, and some intracellular enzymes reactions. Exogenous sources are tobacco smoke, stress, drugs, environmental pollution, xenobiotics, among others [44, 46].

In physiological conditions, antioxidant compounds control ROS levels by an enzymatic system or a non-enzymatic system. The enzymatic system comprises superoxide dismutase (SOD), glutathione peroxidases, and catalase, whereas ascorbic acid (vitamin C), α tocopherol (vitamin E), glutathione, carotenoids, and flavonoids make part of the non-enzymatic system [45]. However, ROS can be maintained at low concentrations because they require different cell processes, including cell proliferation, apoptosis, and gene expression [46]. The oxidant stress is formed due to in balance of ROS production and antioxidant defenses. The cellular lipids, proteins, and DNA can damage due to increase of ROS that can form various stress like diabetes, cancer, neurological disorders, cardiovascular diseases, mutagenesis, and the aging process [25]. For that reason, the improvement of antioxidant-containing foods may help to reduce the harmful effects caused by oxidative damage [45]. Nowadays, researchers are focused on mushroom antioxidant potential due to their high levels of antioxidants like phenolic compounds, polysaccharides, tocopherols, carotenoids, ergosterol, and ascorbic acid are present in the mushroom [47].

In **Table 2**, we have mentioned various mushroom extracts that have abundant antioxidant activity and produced several phenolic compounds. Total phenolic content varied from 5.1 ± 0.5 to 81.33 ± 1.1 mg GAE/g of extract found in *Boletus edulis* and *Boletus griseipurpureus*, respectively. These compounds can act as oxygen scavengers, peroxide decomposes, and free radical inhibitors as per the various researchers [44, 46]. Additionally, few other compounds like pyrogallol, polysaccharides, flavanols, ascorbic acid, and carotenoid compounds are beneficial for antioxidant potential.

Table 2 shows the phenolic and non-phenolic compound detection based on high-performance liquid chromatography (HPLC), nuclear magnetic resonance

Mushroom	Extracts	Method	Type of compound	Others	Reference
Melaleuca sp.	Ethyl acetate, methanol, and aqueous	TPC, TFC, DPPH, ABTS, FRAP, CUPRAC capacity, phospho-molybdenum, and metal chelating assay	Benzoic acid, p-coumaric acid, p-hydroxybenzoic acid, protocatechuic acid, syringic acid, and trans-cinnamic acid	Similar antioxidant ability among *M. cognata* and *M. stridula*	Bahadori et al. [15]
Agaricus silvaticus Schaeff, Hydnum rufescens Pers., and *Meripilus giganteus (Pers.) Karst*	Methanol and ethyl acetate	TPC, TFC, DPPH, ABTS, FRAP, and catalase activity	Phenolic compounds, flavonoids compounds	Only *H. rufescens* demonstrated activity in DPPH and ATBS assay. The ethyl acetate extract displays strongest antioxidant activity in comparison with methanol extract	Garrab et al. [48]
Tuber indicum	Methanol and ethanol	TPC, TFC, DPPH, and ABTS assay	Phenolic compounds, polysaccharides, flavonoids compounds	Variation in the bioactive substances levels and the antioxidant activity depends on *T. indicum* origins	Li et al. [49]
Lentinus squarrosulus	Aqueous	UND	Phytol, octahydropyrrolo, 1,2-alpyrazine, and 3-trifluoroacetoxy-pentadecane	Among the 15 compounds determinate by GC-MS, three of them possess antioxidant activity	Ugbogu et al. [50]
Tricholoma equestre	Aqueous and methanol	TPC and DPPH	UND	Despite methanol extract was richer in phenols than aqueous extract, both are weak antioxidants	Muszyńska et al. [43]
Agaricus bisporus, Flammulina velutipes, Lentinula edodes, and *Agaricus brasiliensis*	UND	TPC, DPPH, ABTS and FRAP assay	Phenolic, gallic acid, protocatechuic acid, catechol, gentisic acid, p-hydroxybenzoic acid, trans-cinnamic acid, p-coumaric acid, ferulic acid, nonphenolic, fumaric acid, and benzoic acid	*Agaricus* brasiliensis showed the higher phenolic content, and antioxidant activity	Bach et al. [29]
Cantharellus cinereus, Clavariadelphus pistillaris, Clitocybe nebularis, Hygrocybe punicea	Methanol, ethanol and aqueous	TPC, DPPH, ABTS, FRAP, TRP, CUPRAC capacity, and FRS activity	Phenolic compounds	Aqueous extracts exerted better antioxidant activity in comparison with methanol and ethanol extracts	Dimitrijevic et al. [51]

Mushroom	Extracts	Method	Type of compound	Others	Reference
Leucoagaricus leucothites	Ethanolic	DPPH, TOS, TAS, and OSI	Phenolic, gallic acid, catechin, and hesperidin	Ethanolic extracts have powerful antioxidant activity suggesting that can be used as an alternative source of antioxidants	Sevindik et al. [42]
Craterellus cornucopioides	Acetone	TPC, DPPH, superoxide anion, scavenging activity, and reducing power	Phenolic acid, gallic acid, p-coumaric acid, chlorogenic acid, caffeic acid, syringic acid, ferulic acid, flavonols, rutin, quercetin, flavan-3-ol, and catechin		Kosanić et al. [30]
Pleurotus levis, Pleurotus ostreatus, Pleurotus pulmonarius, Pleurotus tuberregium	Hydro-alcoholic	TPC, DPPH assay, ORAC capacity, ABTS assay and β-carotene bleaching	Phenolic components	*Pleurotus ostreatus* showed high antioxidant activity. The correlation between TPC and ATBS assay indicated that phenols are the major antioxidant components	Adebayo et al. [52]
Flammulina velutipes, Ganoderma lucidum, Pleurotus ostreatus, Pleurotus pulmonarius	Hexan, ethylacetate, ethanol, methanol, and aqueous	ABTS assay and TEAC	Polysaccharides	*Ganoderma lucidum* possess the higher antioxidant potential in comparison with the other 3 evaluated mushrooms	Chaiharn et al. [32]
Amanita sp., *Lactarius volemus*, *Russula* sp., *Termitomyces* sp., *Tricholoma crissum*, *Volvariella volvácea*, *Astraeus hygrometricus*, *Alpova trappei*, *Auricularia auricula, Cantharellus cibarius, Cra Craterellus aureus, and Lentinus* sp.	Methanol	TPC, TFC, DPPH, and FRAP	Flavonols, quercetin, quercetin-3-O-rutinoside, myricetin, kaempferol, flavan-3-ols, catechin, epicatechin, flavanone, and naringenin	*T. clypeatus* and *V. volvacea* show the highest antioxidant activity and the highest concentrations of phenolic compounds. Despite, these two mushrooms can be included in the diet, it is needed more studies to determine if it can be used as a food supplement	Butkhup et al. [53]

Mushroom	Extracts	Method	Type of compound	Others	Reference
Macrocybe lobayensis	Hydro ethanol	TPC, DPPH assay, ABTS assay, superoxide radical, hydroxyl radical quenching chelating ability of metal ion, reducing power, and TAC	Ferulic acid, cinnamic acid, pyrogallol, flavonoid, ascorbic acid, β-carotene, and lycopene	The obtained hydro-ethanol extract was enriched with bioactive compounds and exhibited strong antioxidant potentiality	Khatua et al. [54]
Boletus edulis, Boletus pinophilus, Boletus aureus, Armillaria mellea, Tuber aestivum, Lactarius piperatus, Lactarius deliciosus, Pleurotus eryngii, Ramaria botrytis, and *Russula virescens*	Ethanol	DPPH assay, chelating activity, reducing power, and inhibition of lipid peroxidation	Caffeic acid, gallic acid, 3,4 and 2,5 dihydroxybenzoic, cinnamic acid, phenols, flavonoids, flavonols, anthocyanins, proanthocyanidins, ascorbic acid, lycopeneand, and β-carotene	Polysaccharide compound was correlated with DPPH assay activity. Phenolic compounds were correlated with the reducing power, and the inhibition of lipid peroxidation	Vamanu [55]
Pleurotus ostreatus	UND	DPPH and ABTS assay	Three them were new amino acid derivatives	These three new compounds: (1) $C_{12}H_{14}N_2O_4$, (2) $C_9H_{16}N_2O_4$, and (3) $C_{12}H_{12}N_4O_3$ have comparable antioxidant activity with that of the standard compound	Lu et al. [56]
Agaricus lanipes	Methanol	TPC, TAC, TOS, LOOHs, and TFS	UND	This is the first report of the antioxidant activity of *Agaricus lanipes*	Kaygusuz et al. [39]
Agaricus bisporus and *Ganoderma lucidum*	Aqueous	DPPH assay	Flavonoids and carboxylic acids	*A. bisporus* silver nanoparticles possess the highest antioxidant ability	Sriramulu and Sumathi [57]
Agaricus lanipes	Methanol	TPC, TAC, TOS, LOOHs, and TFS	UND	This is the first report of the antioxidant activity of *Agaricus lanipes*	Kaygusuz et al. [39]
Ramaria subalpine	Methanol	TPC, TFC, ascorbic acid content, ß-carotene and lycopene content, DPPH, ferrous ion chelating, and reducing power	Pyrogallol	This edible mushroom showed potentiality in the antioxidant activity assays. Otherwise, phenolic compounds were the major bioactive component founded	Acharya et al. [58]

Mushroom	Extracts	Method	Type of compound	Others	Reference
Agaricus campestris and *Boletus edulis*	Methanol	Total soluble phenolic compounds, TPC, DPPH assay, and reducing power	Phenolic compounds	Despite *B. edulis* possess higher antioxidant activity than *A. campestris*, both can be an alternative for antioxidant sources	Kosanić et al. [59]
Boletus griseipurpureus	Dichloromethane and methanol	TPC, DPPH, oxygen radical absorbance, ORAC, and ABTS assay	Phenolic compounds	*Boletus griseipurpureus* extracts showed similar antioxidant activity to other *Boletus* species as previous studies	Sudjaroen and Thongkao [60]

UND-undetermined; TPC-total phenolic content; TFC-total flavonoids content; FRAP-ferric reducing antioxidant power; CUPRAC-cupric reducing antioxidant capacity; TRP-total reducing power; FRS-determination of free radical scavenging; TOS-total oxidant status; TAS-total antioxidant status; OSI-oxidative stress index; TEAC-trolox equivalent antioxidant capacity; ORAC-oxygen radical absorbance capacity; TAC-total antioxidant capacity; LOOHs-lipid hydroperoxides; TFS-total free sulfhydryl group.

Table 2.
Studies on antioxidant activity in edible mushroom.

(NMR) analysis, chromatographic method or gas chromatography–mass spectrometry (GC–MS). Moreover, **Table 2** described that the different kinds of mushrooms could be used to determine the antioxidant activity potential in several ways, such as 1,1-diphenyl-2-picrylhydrazyl (DPPH), 2,2′-azinobis-(3-ethylbenzthiazoline-6-sulphonate (ABTS), and ferric-reducing antioxidant power (FRAP). Further, Sriramulu and Sumathi [57] demonstrated that extract of edible *Agaricus bisporus* and wild *Ganoderma lucidum* mushroom was used to synthesize silver nanoparticles that showed photocatalytic activity and biological activities such as in vitro antioxidant activity, anti-inflammatory activity, and antimicrobial activity against bacterial pathogens such as *E. coli* and *S. aureus*. Garrab et al. [48] reported that ethyl acetate extract of *Agaricus silvaticus* Schaeff., *Hydnum rufescens* Pers., and *Meripilus giganteus* (Pers.) Karst. exhibited antioxidant and anticholinesterase activity. Interestingly, ethyl acetate extract of *Hydnum rufescens Pers.* indicated the highest antioxidant activity in DPPH and catalase potential. Recently, many researches are focusing on extracting the compound like chitosan and chitosan + procyanidin obtained from a mushroom that can be used to coat the blueberries, which revealed the higher antioxidant potential as compared to no coated berries [61]. Similarly, Velez et al. [62] reported that AA-loaded chitosan/tripolyphosphate nanoaggregates obtained from mushrooms, which can be useful to coat the fresh-cut mushrooms that displayed significant antioxidant activity. Moreover, some studies had reported that antioxidant activity, total phenolic compounds, and total flavonoid compounds increased in tarhana and bread after the addition of *Morchella conica*, *Ramaria flava,* and *Agaricus bisporus* powder [16, 17].

In addition, some researchers are investigated to study the antiangiogenic potential to prevent neurological disorders and hepatoprotective properties. A p-terphenyl compound is derived from two edible mushrooms that showed the anticancer effect to averts vascular endothelial growth factor with the presence of antioxidant and anti-inflammatory activity [63]. Few researchers reported that benzoic acid derivative compounds such as be p-hydroxybenzoic, protocatechuic, gallic, gentisic, homogentisic, vanillic, 5-sulphosalicylic, syringic, veratric, and vanillin obtained from diverse types of much room such as *Phellinus rimosus, Ganoderma lucidum, Ganoderma tsugae, Coriolus versicolor, Lentinus edodes, Volvariella volvacea, Termitomyces heimii, Helvella crispa, Termitomyces tylerance, Lactarius sanguifluus, Morchella conica, Termitomyces mummiformis, Pleurotus sajor-caju, Termitomyces schimperi, Lentinus squarrulosus, Boletus edulis, Pleurotus djamor, Macrolepiota procera, Cantharellus clavatus, Morchella angusticeps,* and *Termitomyces microcarpus* [25]. Recently, a few different polyphenols like curcumin, resveratrol, and quercetin showed pro-oxidant activity that can act as photosensitizers to produce $1O_2$ as per Lagunes and Trigos [64]. Additionally, Li et al. [65] reported that the aqueous extract of *Amanita caesarea* was estimated in an L-glutamic acid to induce the HT22 cell apoptosis model. In contrast, D-galactose and $AlCl_3$ have improved Alzheimer's disease (AD) in the mice model to prevent neurogenerative diseases. One of the interesting studies Chen et al. [66] explored is that polysaccharides isolated from *Grifola frondosa* could be used to improve memory impairment in aged rats by increasing total antioxidant capacity, glutathione peroxidase activity, superoxide dismutase activity, and catalase activity. Dong et al. [67] indicated that enzyme-assisted *M. esculenta* polysaccharide enhances hepatic antioxidant enzymes that can decrease the amount of lipid peroxidation in mice models.

5. Conclusion and concluding remarks

Mushroom is widely useful as food supplements and suitable for all the age groups due to their high content of protein, dietary fiber, vitamins, and mineral. Moreover, they contain various bioactive molecules such as polysaccharides, terpenoids, glycoproteins, antimicrobial compounds, antioxidants, etc. that can play a major role in the treatment of numerous diseases like improving immune strength, decreasing the cancer level in the body, reducing blood sugar level, inhibiting the multidrug resistant bacterial pathogen, and many more. In this review, we have focused on antioxidant and antimicrobial activity of edible and non-edible mushrooms all over the world and their uses. We have found that few of the mushroom are producing wide variety of bioactive phenolic compounds such as pyrogallol, polysaccharides, flavanols, ascorbic acid, and carotenoid compounds that can be used to control various diseases like antitumor, antimicrobial, antioxidant and anti-hypertensive, hypocholesterolemic, and hepatoprotective activity. Mushrooms like *Agaricus silvaticus Schaeff, Hydnum rufescens Pers., Meripilus giganteus (Pers.) Karst., Termitomyces sp. Tricholoma crissum, Volvariella volvácea, Astraeus hygrometricus, Alpova trappei, Auricularia auricula, Cantharellus cibarius, Cra Craterellus aureus, Lentinus sp.*, etc. showed significant antioxidant activity and produced various compounds that detected by HPLC, GC-MS, and NMR spectroscopy as presented in the tables. Further, different solvent extracts of *Xerocomus ichnussanus, Boletus lupinus, Flammulina velutipes, Phellinus igniarius, Sarcodon imbricatus, Tricholoma aurantium, Agaricus bisporus, Pleurotus ostreatus, and Lentinula edodes* exhibited potent antimicrobial activity against Gram-positive and Gram-negative bacteria as shown in the table. It can be concluded that mushroom has high therapeutic potential that could be used for the development of new formulations, which can be beneficial for new nutraceutical products. Hence, new methods should be used to isolate novel compounds from different mushrooms that can be used for the deterrence and decrease of several diseases.

Acknowledgements

Authors are thankful to the DGAPA, UNAM grants IN202216 and IN205519, for their grateful support in completion of the book chapter.

Conflict of interest

The authors declare that no conflict of interest for this publication.

Author details

Maria Paula Gómez Román[1†], Nathalia Badillo Mantilla[1†], Sergio Andrés Carreño Flórez[1], Surajit De Mandal[2], Ajit Kumar Passari[1*†], Beatriz Ruiz-Villáfan[1], Romina Rodríguez-Sanoja[1] and Sergio Sánchez[1*]

1 Instituto de Investigaciones Biomédicas, Universidad Nacional Autónoma De México, Ciudad de México, Mexico

2 College of Agriculture, South China Agricultural University, Guangzhou, P.R. China

*Address all correspondence to: ajit.passari22@iibiomedicas.unam.mx and sersan@biomedicas.unam.mx

† These authors contributed equally to this work.

References

[1] Pommerville JC. Fundamentals of Microbiology. Burlington, Mass: Jones and Bartlett Publishers; 2014

[2] Hawksworth DL. Mushrooms: The extent of the unexplored potential. International Journal of Medicinal Mushrooms. 2001;**3**:333-337

[3] Ukwuru MU, Muritala A, Eze LU. Edible and non-edible wild mushrooms: Nutrition, toxicity and strategies for recognition. Journal of Clinical Nutrition and Metabolism. 2018;**2**

[4] Jayachandran M, Xiao J, Xu B. A critical review on health promoting benefits of edible mushrooms through gut microbiota. International Journal of Molecular Sciences. 2017;**18**(9). pii: E1934. DOI: 10.3390/ijms18091934

[5] Mhanda F, Kadhila N, Ueitele I. Minerals and trace elements in domesticated Namibian Ganoderma species. African Journal of Biotechnology. 2015;**14**(48):3216-3218. DOI: 10.5897/ajb2015.14573

[6] Singh BP, Chhakchhuak L, Passari AK, editors. Biology of Macrofungi. Switzerland: Springer International Publisher; 2018. DOI: 10.1007/978-3-030-02622-6

[7] Lallawmsanga, Passari AK, Mishra VK, Leo VV, Singh BP, Meyyappan GV, et al. Antimicrobial potential, identification and phylogenetic affiliation of wild mushrooms from two sub-tropical semi-evergreen indian forest ecosystems. PLoS One. 2016;**11**(11):e0166368. DOI: 10.1371/journal.pone.0166368

[8] Akabanda F, Owusu-Kwarteng J, Tano-Debrah K, Glover R, Nielsen LK, et al. Taxonomic and molecular characterization of lactic acid bacteria and yeasts in nunu, a Ghanaian fermented milk product. Food Microbiology. 2013;**34**:277-283

[9] Pathirage KP, Yunman L. Mushrooms as a functional food mediator in preventing and ameliorating diabetes. Functional Foods in Health and Disease. 2011;**4**:161-171

[10] Turkoglu A, Kivrak I, Mercan N, Duru ME, Gezer K, Turkoglu H. Antioxidant and antimicrobial activities of *Morchella conica* Pers. African Journal of Biotechnology. 2006;**5**:1146-1150

[11] Aziz T, Mehmet ED, Nazime AM. Antioxidant and antimicrobial activity of *Russula delica* Fr: An Edi wild Mus. European Journal of Anal Chemistry. 2007;**2**:64-67

[12] Gaglio R, Guarcello R, Venturella G, Palazzolo E, Francesca N, Moschetti G, et al. Microbiological, chemical and sensory aspects of bread supplemented with different percentages of the culinary mushroom *Pleurotus eryngii* in powder form. International Journal of Food Science & Technology. 2018;**54**(4):1197-1205. DOI: 10.1111/ijfs.13997

[13] Balaji P, Madhanraj R, Ravi Kumar K, Maya MR, Illuri R, Venkatakrishna K, et al. Evaluation of anti-microbial and anti-haemolytic activity of edible basidiomycetes mushroom fungi. Journal of Drug Delivery and Therapeutics. 2019;**9**(1):132-135. DOI: 10.22270/jddt.v9i1.2277

[14] Valverde ME, Hernandez-Perez T, Paredes-Lopez O. Edible mushrooms: Improving human health and promoting quality life. International Journal of Microbiology. 2015;**2015**:376387. DOI: 10.1155/2015/376387

[15] Bahadori MB, Sarikurkcu C, Yalcin OU, Cengiz M, Gungor H. Metal

concentration, phenolics profiling, and antioxidant activity of two wild edible Melanoleuca mushrooms (*M. cognata* and *M. stridula*). Microchemical Journal. 2019;**150**:104172

[16] Eker T, Bozok F. Effect of edible mushroom powder on antioxidant activity of Tarhana. Indian Journal of Pharmaceutical Education and Research. 2019;**51**:S268-S270

[17] Zhang Y, Ruan C, Cheng Z, Zhou Y, Liang J. Mixolab behavior, quality attributes and antioxidant capacity of breads incorporated with *Agaricus bisporus*. Journal of Food Science and Technology. 2019;**56**:1-9

[18] Boa E. Wild Edible Fungi: A Global Overview of their Use and Importance to People. Non-wood Forest Products. Rome: Food & Agriculture Org; 2004

[19] Kaul T. Conservation of mushroom biodiversity. In: Mushroom Biology and Biotechnology (388). Solan: Mushroom Society of India; 2007

[20] Willey JM, Sherwood L, Woolverton CJ, Prescott LM, Willey JM. Prescott's Microbiology. New York: McGraw-Hil; 2011

[21] Carlile MJ, Watkinson SC, Gooday GW. The Fungi. London: Academic, San Diego; 2001

[22] Borges A, Ferreira C, Saavedra MJ, Simoes M. Antibacterial activity and mode of action of ferulic and gallic acids against pathogenic bacteria. Microbial Drug Resistance. 2013;**19**(4):256-265. DOI: 10.1089/mdr.2012.0244

[23] World Health Organization (WHO), 2013. Global strategy for containment of antimicrobial resistance. WHO/CDS/CSR/DRS/2001.2

[24] Ashbolt NJ, Amézquita A, Backhaus T, Borriello P, Brandt KK, Collignon P, et al. Human health risk assessment (HHRA) for environmental development and transfer of antibiotic resistance. Environmental Health Perspectives. 2013;**121**(9):993-1001. DOI: 10.1289/ehp.1206316

[25] Ferreira ICFR, Barros L, Abreu RMV. Antioxidants in wild mushrooms. Current Medicinal Chemistry. 2009;**16**:1543-1156

[26] Lallawmsanga, Leo VV, Passari AK, Muniraj IK, Uthandi S, Hashem A, et al. Elevated levels of laccase synthesis by *Pleurotus pulmonarius* BPSM10 and its potential as a dye decolorizing agent. Saudi Journal of Biological Sciences. 2018;**26**(3):464-468

[27] Mishra VK, Passari AK, Leo VV, Singh BP. Molecular diversity and detection of endophytic fungi based on their antimicrobial biosynthetic genes. In: Singh BP, Gupta VK, editors. Molecular Markers in Mycology, Fungal Biology. Switzerland: Springer International Publisher; 2016. pp. 1-35. DOI: 10.1007/978-3-319-34106-4_1

[28] Alves MJ, Ferreira IC, Dias J, Teixeira V, Martins A, Pintado M. A review on antimicrobial activity of mushroom (Basidiomycetes) extracts and isolated compounds. Planta Medica. 2012;**78**(16):1707-1718. DOI: 10.1055/s-0032-1315370

[29] Bach F, Zielinski AAF, Helm CV, Maciel GM, Pedro AC, Stafussa AP, et al. Bio compounds of edible mushrooms: in vitro antioxidant and antimicrobial activities. Food Science and Technology. 2019;**107**:214-220. DOI: 10.1016/j.lwt.2019.03.017

[30] Kosanić M, Ranković B, Stanojković T, Radović-Jakovljević M, Ćirić A, Grujičić D, et al. Craterellus cornucopioides edible mushroom as source of biologically active compounds. Natural Product Communications. 2019;**14**(5):1-6. DOI: 10.1177/1934578x19843610

[31] Varshney J, Ooi JH, Jayarao BM, Albert I, Fisher J, Smith RL, et al. White button mushrooms increase microbial diversity and accelerate the resolution of *Citrobacter rodentium* infection in mice. The Journal of Nutrition. 2013;**143**(4):526-532. DOI: 10.3945/jn.112.171355

[32] Chaiharn M, Phutdhawong WS, Amornlerdpison D, Phutdhawong W. Antibacterial, antioxidant properties and bioactive compounds of Thai cultivated mushroom extracts against food-borne bacterial strains. Chiang Mai Journal of Science. 2018;**45**:1713-1727

[33] Nikolovska D, Atanasova N, Amedi H, Veleska D, Ivanova E, Karadelev M, et al. Screening of antibacterial and antifungal activities of selected Macedonian wild mushrooms. Zbornik Matice srpske za prirodne nauke. 2013;**124**:333-340. DOI: 10.2298/zmspn1324333n

[34] Li S, Shah NP. Antioxidant and antibacterial activities of sulphated polysaccharides from *Pleurotus eryngii* and *Streptococcus thermophilus* ASCC 1275. Food Chemistry. 2014;**165**:262-270. DOI: 10.1016/j.foodchem.2014.05.110

[35] Matijasevic D, Pantic M, Raskovic B, Pavlovic V, Duvnjak D, Sknepnek A, et al. The antibacterial activity of *Coriolus versicolor* methanol extract and its effect on Ultrastructural changes of *Staphylococcus aureus* and *Salmonella* Enteritidis. Frontiers in Microbiology. 2016;7:1226. DOI: 10.3389/fmicb.2016.01226

[36] Kosanić M, Rankovic B, Rancic A, Stanojkovic T. Evaluation of metal concentration and antioxidant, antimicrobial, and anticancer potentials of two edible mushrooms *Lactarius deliciosus* and *Macrolepiota procera*. Journal of Food and Drug Analysis. 2016;**24**(3):477-484. DOI: 10.1016/j.jfda.2016.01.008

[37] Taofiq O, Heleno SA, Calhelha RC, Alves MJ, Barros L, Barreiro MF, et al. Development of mushroom-based cosmeceutical formulations with anti-inflammatory, anti-tyrosinase, antioxidant, and antibacterial properties. Molecules. 2016;**21**(10). pii: E1372. DOI: 10.3390/molecules21101372

[38] Shameem N, Kamili AN, Ahmad M, Masoodi FA, Parray JA. Antimicrobial activity of crude fractions and morel compounds from wild edible mushrooms of north western Himalaya. Microbial Pathogenesis. 2017;**105**:356-360. DOI: 10.1016/j.micpath.2017.03.005

[39] Kaygusuz O, Kaygusuz M, Dodurga Y, Secme M, Herken EN, Gezer K. Assessment of the antimicrobial, antioxidant and cytotoxic activities of the wild edible mushroom Agaricus lanipes (F.H. Moller & Jul. Schaff.) Hlavacek. Cytotechnology. 2017;**69**(1):135-144. DOI: 10.1007/s10616-016-0045-4

[40] Mohanarji S, Dharmalingam S, Anandarajagopal, Kalusalingam. Screening of *Lignosus rhinocerus* extracts as antimicrobial agents against selected human pathogens. Journal of Pharmaceutical and Biomedical Sciences. 2012;**18**(18):11

[41] Nallathamby N, Phan CW, Seow SL, Baskaran A, Lakshmanan H, Abd Malek SN, et al. A status review of the bioactive activities of tiger milk mushroom *Lignosus rhinocerotis* (Cooke) Ryvarden. Frontiers in Pharmacology. 2017;**8**:998. DOI: 10.3389/fphar.2017.00998

[42] Sevindik M, Rasul A, Hussain G, Anwar H, Zahoor MK, Sarfraz I, et al. Determination of anti-oxidative, anti-microbial activity and heavy metal contents of *Leucoagaricus leucothites*. Pakistan Journal of Pharmaceutical Sciences. 2018;**31**:2163-2168

[43] Muszyńska B, Kała K, Radović J, Sułkowska-Ziaja K, Krakowska A, Gdula-Argasińska J, et al. Study of biological activity of Tricholoma equestre fruiting bodies and their safety for human. European Food Research and Technology. 2018;**244**(12):2255-2264. DOI: 10.1007/s00217-018-3134-0

[44] Sánchez C. Reactive oxygen species and antioxidant properties from mushrooms. Synthetic and Systems Biotechnology. 2017;**2**:13-22

[45] Khatua S, Paul S, Acharya K. Mushroom as the potential source of new generation of antioxidant: A review. Research Journal of Pharmacy and Technology. 2013;**6**:496-505

[46] Kozarski M, Klaus A, Jakovljevic D, Todorovic N, Vunduk J, Petrović P, et al. Antioxidants of edible mushrooms. Molecules. 2015;**20**:19489-19525

[47] Kalaras MD, Richie JP, Calcagnotto A, Beelman RB. Mushrooms: A rich source of the antioxidants ergothioneine and glutathione. Food Chemistry. 2017;**233**:429-433

[48] Garrab M, Edziri H, El Mokni R, Mastouri M, Mabrouk H, Douki W. Phenolic composition, antioxidant and anticholinesterase properties of the three mushrooms *Agaricus silvaticus* Schaeff., *Hydnum rufescens* Pers. and *Meripilus giganteus* (Pers.) karst. in Tunisia. South African Journal of Science. 2019;**124**:359-363

[49] Li J, Liang H, Qiao P, Su K, Liu P, Guo S, et al. Chemical composition and antioxidant activity of tuber indicum from different geographical regions of China. Chemistry & Biodiversity. 2019;**16**:e1800609

[50] Ugbogu EA, Akubugwo IE, Ude VC, Gilbert J, Ekeanyanwu B. Toxicological evaluation of phytochemical characterized aqueous extract of wild dried *Lentinus squarrosulus* (Mont.) mushroom in rats. Toxicological Research. 2019;**35**:181-190

[51] Dimitrijevic MV, Mitic VD, Nikolic JS, Djordjevic AS, Mutic JJ, Jovanovic VPS, et al. First report about mineral content, fatty acids composition and biological activities of four wild edible mushrooms. Chemistry & Biodiversity. 2019;**16**:e1800492

[52] Adebayo EA, Martinez-Carrera D, Morales P, et al. Comparative study of antioxidant and antibacterial properties of the edible mushrooms *Pleurotus levis*, *P. ostreatus*, *P. pulmonarius* and *P. tuber-regium*. International Journal of Food Science & Technology. 2018;**53**:1316-1330

[53] Butkhup L, Samappito W, Jorjong S. Evaluation of bioactivities and phenolic contents of wild edible mushroom from northeastern Thailand. Food Science and Biotechnology. 2018;**27**:193-202

[54] Khatua S, Ghosh S, Acharya K. Antioxidant properties and metabolites profiling of polyphenol-rich fraction from a folk mushroom, *Macrocybe lobayensis*, using different extractant. International Journal of Research in Pharmaceutical Sciences. 2018;**10**:564-571

[55] Vamanu E. Bioactive capacity of some Romanian wild edible mushrooms consumed mainly by local communities. Natural Product Research. 2018;**32**:440-443

[56] Lu XJ, Feng BM, Chen SF, Zhao D, Chen G, Wang HF, et al. Three new amino acid derivatives from edible mushroom *Pleurotus ostreatus*. Journal of Asian Natural Products Research. 2017;**19**:1160-1171

[57] Sriramulu M, Sumathi S. Photocatalytic, antioxidant, antibacterial and anti-inflammatory activity of silver nanoparticles

synthesised using forest and edible mushroom. Advances in Natural Sciences: Nanoscience and Nanotechnology. 2017;**8**:1-9

[58] Acharya K, Das K, Paloi S, Dutta AK, Hembrom ME, Somanjana K, et al. Exploring a novel edible mushroom *Ramaria subalpina*: Chemical characterization and antioxidant activity. Pharmacognosy Journal. 2017;**9**:30-34

[59] Kosanić M, Ranković B, Rančić A, Stanojković T. Evaluation of metal contents and bioactivity of two edible mushrooms *Agaricus campestris* and boletus edulis. Emirates Journal of Food and Agriculture. 2017;**29**:98-103

[60] Sudjaroen Y, Thongkao K. Screening of nutritive values, in vitro antioxidant, anticancer and antimicrobial activities from boletus griseipurpureus corner. International Journal of Green Pharmacy. 2017;**11**:74-80

[61] Mannozzi C, Tylewicz U, Chinnici F, Siroli L, Rocculi P, Dalla Rosa M, et al. Effects of chitosan-based coatings enriched with procyanidin by-product on quality of fresh blueberries during storage. Food Chemistry. 2018;**251**:18-24

[62] Velez MEV, da Luz JMR, da Silva MCS, Cardoso WS, Lopes LS, Vieira NA, et al. Production of bioactive compounds by the mycelial growth of Pleurotus djamor in whey powder enriched with selenium. LWT. 2019;**114**:108376

[63] Sonowal H, Shukla K, Kota S, Saxena A, Ramana KV. Vialinin a, an edible mushroom-derived p-Terphenyl antioxidant, prevents VEGF-induced neovascularization In vitro and In vivo. Oxidative Medicine and Cellular Longevity. 2018;**2018**:1-10

[64] Lagunes I, Trigos A. Photo-oxidation of ergosterol: Indirect detection of antioxidants photosensitizers or quenchers of singlet oxygen. Journal of Photochemistry and Photobiology B. 2015;**145**:30-34

[65] Li Z, Chen X, Lu W, Zhang S, Guan X, Li Z, et al. Anti-oxidative stress activity is essential for Amanita caesarea mediated neuroprotection on glutamate-induced apoptotic HT22 cells and an Alzheimer's disease mouse model. International Journal of Molecular Sciences. 2017;**18**:E1623

[66] Chen Z, Tang Y, Liu A, Jin X, Zhu J, Lu X. Oral administration of *Grifola frondosa* polysaccharides improves memory impairment in aged rats via antioxidant action. Molecular Nutrition & Food Research. 2017;**61**:1700313

[67] Dong Y, Qi Y, Liu M, Song X, Zhang C, Jiao X, et al. Antioxidant, anti-hyperlipidemia and hepatic protection of enzyme-assisted *Morehella esculenta* polysaccharide. International Journal of Biological Macromolecules. 2018;**120**:1490-1499

Chapter 2

Edible Mushroom: Nutritional Properties, Potential Nutraceutical Values, and Its Utilisation in Food Product Development

Lee-Hoon Ho, Noroul Asyikeen Zulkifli and Thuan-Chew Tan

Abstract

Edible mushrooms are an excellent source of proteins, minerals, polysaccharides, unsaturated fatty acids, and secondary metabolites. Numerous studies have provided evidence for the protective effects of edible mushrooms against various chronic diseases. In this review, details on the compositions and nutritional values of edible mushrooms were discussed. Furthermore, bioactive compounds such as polyphenolic compounds and antioxidant capacity of edible mushrooms, as well as the application of these edible mushrooms as potential therapeutic agents, were covered. This chapter also endeavoured to review the recent progress on the potential utilisation of edible mushrooms in the development of functional food products and its effects on the nutritional, physical, and organoleptic properties of the developed food products. Based on the recent socioeconomic trends, the substitution of edible mushroom as an essential source of functional ingredients in food products could become a natural adjuvant for the prevention and alleviation of several lifestyle-related diseases. This information could be beneficial for the development of food products with health functionalities, which are of great interest to the medical nutrition industry, which is an industry that emerged from the convergence between the food and pharma industries.

Keywords: edible mushroom, nutritional compositions, functional properties, nutraceutical properties, therapeutic values, food product quality

1. Introduction

Mycophagy describes the practice of eating mushrooms. This practice can be dated back to ancient times, whereby wild edible mushrooms were collected and consumed. Mushrooms are an excellent source of vitamins, e.g. B vitamins and vitamin D [1], and minerals, e.g. phosphorus, magnesium, selenium, copper, and potassium [2], and are also rich in dietary fibre, chitin and β-glucans [3]. Humans have, for centuries, consumed mushrooms not only for nutrition [4, 5] and taste [6] but also for their healing properties [7]. Numerous studies have shown that mushrooms are a rich source of bioactive compounds, e.g. phenolic and flavonoid compounds, that exert antioxidant properties, and these could be beneficial to human health [8–12]. Mushrooms could help in reducing the risk of diseases, such as Parkinson's, Alzheimer's, hypertension, stroke, and cancer, as well as act as an antibacterial, immune system enhancer, and cholesterol-lowering agents [13].

Due to the numerous reports and findings on the health benefits of mushrooms to humans, studies on the use of mushrooms as a bioactive ingredient in functional food products have gained attention from the scientific community. Mushrooms are converted into powder before incorporated into food products, such as bread, muffins, pasta, patties, and snacks, to increase the nutritional quality of these products [14–18]. With the introduction of processed food products incorporated with mushrooms, this further expands the popularity of mushrooms among consumers. On average, consumers consumed about 5 kg of mushrooms per person per year, and this number is expected to continue to increase as consumers become more aware of the healthful benefits of incorporating mushrooms in their diet [19].

For the last 10 years, from 2008 to 2017, the global production of mushrooms and truffles grew from 6.90 to 10.24 million metric tons [20] (**Figure 1**). Based on the latest statistic report from the Food and Agriculture Organization of the United Nations, in 2017, China (7.87 million metric tons, contributed almost 77% of world production), the United States (0.42 million metric tons), the Netherlands (0.30 million metric tons), Poland (0.30 million metric tons), and Spain (0.16 million metric tons) were reported as the top 5 mushroom and truffle producers in the world. As the demand for edible mushrooms increases and the amount of wild edible mushrooms shrinks, edible mushroom cultivation is becoming an important agriculture sector.

The most cultivated edible mushroom worldwide is *Agaricus bisporus* (common mushroom) followed by *Lentinus edodes* (shiitake mushroom), *Pleurotus* spp. (in particular oyster mushroom), and *Flammulina velutipes* (enoki mushroom) [3, 13, 21]. Moisture content varies around 90% for raw mushrooms. Typically, mushrooms are low in fat and contain useful minerals and B vitamins. Though mushrooms are not energy-providing foods, mushrooms are a substantially better source of nutrition than is often assumed [22].

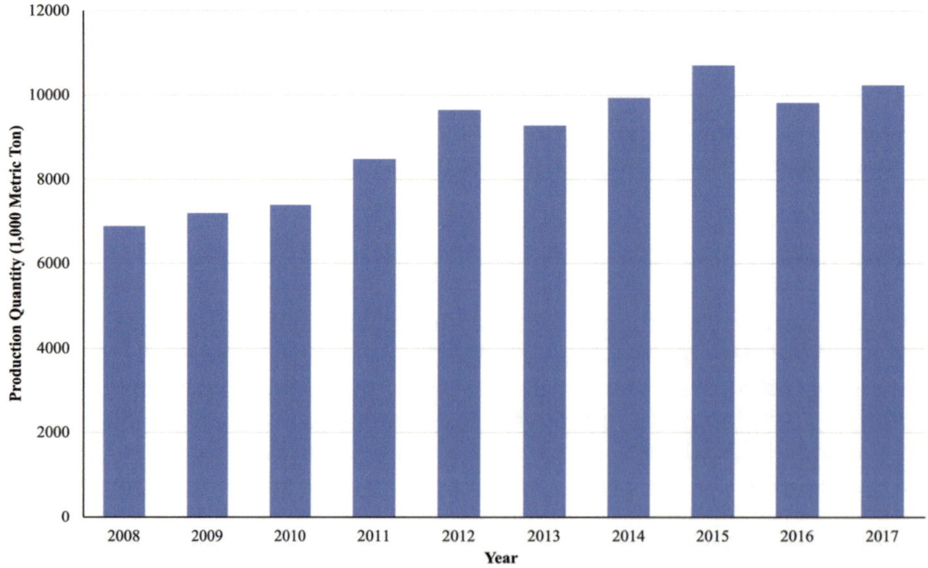

Figure 1.
Growth in world mushrooms and truffles production, 2008–2017. Source: [20].

2. Nutritional compositions

Edible mushrooms possess high nutritional value, especially protein and carbohydrates. Besides, edible mushrooms have also been described as a rich source of minerals and vitamins [23, 24]. The mean nutrient values for these raw mushrooms [25] are presented in **Table 1**. Han et al. [24] studied the quality properties of powder processed from oyster mushroom, a variety of *Pleurotus sajor-caju* (PSC). Their results showed PSC powder had a high content of carbohydrate (60.47 g/100 g), resulting in 451.60 cal/g calorie. According to Samsudin and Abdullah [21], mushrooms provide both digestible carbohydrates (i.e. trehalose, mannitol, glycogen, and glucose) and non-digestible carbohydrate (i.e. mannans, chitin, and β-glucan). Later, both these carbohydrates form the larger portion of the total carbohydrates. Aremu et al. [26] reported that the calculated metabolisable energy values in *Ganoderma* spp. (1476.7 kJ/100 g) and in *Hebeloma mesophaeum* (1513.5 kJ/100 g) indicate that both varieties of mushrooms are concentrated sources of energy and compared favourably to cereals in terms of their energy values.

Nutrient	Common mushroom	Shiitake mushroom	Oyster mushroom	Enoki mushroom
Moisture (g/100 g)	92.45	89.74	89.18	88.34
Energy (kcal/100 g)	22	34	33	37
Protein (g/100 g)	3.09	2.24	3.31	2.66
Fat (g/100 g)	0.34	0.49	0.41	0.29
Ash (g/100 g)	0.85	0.73	1.01	0.91
Carbohydrate (g/100 g)	3.26	6.79	6.09	7.81
Dietary fibre (g/100 g)	1.0	2.5	2.3	2.7
Ergosterol (mg/100 g)	56	85	64	36
Calcium (mg/100 g)	3	2	3	0
Copper (mg/100 g)	0.32	0.14	0.24	0.11
Iron (mg/100 g)	0.5	0.41	1.33	1.15
Magnesium (mg/100 g)	9	20	18	16
Manganese (mg/100 g)	0.05	0.23	0.11	0.08
Phosphorus (mg/100 g)	86	112	120	105
Potassium (mg/100 g)	318	304	420	359
Selenium (μg/100 g)	9.3	5.7	2.6	2.2
Sodium (mg/100 g)	5	9	18	3
Zinc (mg/100 g)	0.52	1.03	0.77	0.65
Thiamin (mg/100 g)	0.081	0.015	0.125	0.225
Riboflavin (mg/100 g)	0.40	0.22	0.35	0.20
Niacin (mg/100 g)	3.61	3.88	4.96	7.03
Pantothenic acid (mg/100 g)	1.50	1.50	1.29	1.35
Pyridoxine (mg/100 g)	0.10	0.29	0.11	0.10

Source: USDA [25].

Table 1.
Mean nutrient content of raw mushrooms per 100 g edible portion.

On the other hand, Han et al. [24] reported that PSC contained 22.4 g/100 g protein, 56.99 g/100 g dietary fibre (i.e. 56.99 g/100 g total dietary fibre, 48.79 g/100 g insoluble dietary fibre, and 8.20 g/100 g soluble dietary fibre), 7.79 g/100 g ash, and 3.32 g/100 g β-glucan but has low amount of sucrose (0.19 g/100 g) and crude fat (2.30 g/100 g). According to Elleuch et al. [27], polysaccharides especially dietary fibres are the most important active compounds among others. Hence, several medicinal and pharmacological properties of PSC are believed to be associated with dietary fibre which can provide functional properties.

It is interesting to note that different parts of mushroom, the cap, stalk, or cap with a stalk of oyster mushroom (*Pleurotus ostreatus*), an edible mushroom, presented different proximate compositions [28]. The results showed that the stalk of mushrooms had the highest moisture content (6.33 g/100 g) than the other parts of mushrooms, whereas the cap showed the least moisture content (3.48 g/100 g). In addition, there was a noticeable difference in their protein content, 34.19 g/100 g of the cap, 20.96 g/100 g of a stalk, and 30.48 g/100 g of the cap with a stalk. Cruz-Solorio et al. [29] reported that the fruit body of *Pleurotus ostreatus* has significant nutritional values and highly valuable protein concentrates. Protein fractionation revealed that globulin had the highest proportion with 47.31% present in the cap, 23.31% in stalk, and 44.65% present in cap with a stalk, while albumin varied between 3.29 and 4.18% in cap, stalk, and cap with a stalk [28]. Moreover, the cap, stalk, and stalk with a cap were reported to have 3.14 g/100 g, 7.53 g/100 g, and 8.12 g/100 g, respectively, of crude fibre. The ash content was between 5.30 and 8.24 g/100 g for all parts of the mushroom; the fat content was 1.48 g/100 g, 1.55 g/100 g, and 1.5 g/100 g for the stalk, cap, and stalk with the cap, respectively. Carbohydrate content ranges between 51.94 and 61.77 g/100 g [28].

In another study by Kayode et al. [23], they found that the proximate compositions of exotic oyster mushroom grown on *Gmelina* wood waste and indigenous wild species of oyster mushroom (i.e. PSC) have 7.00 g/100 g and 7.15 g/100 g moisture, 19.30 g/100 g and 25.24 g/100 g protein, 7.24 g/100 g and 6.65 g/100 g crude fat, 7.47 g/100 g and 7.05 g/100 g crude fibre, 7.13 g/100 g and 8.25 g/100 g ash, and 51.86 g/100 g and 45.66 g/100 g total carbohydrate, respectively. This study concluded that oyster mushroom grown on *Gmelina* wood waste is favourably compared with the wild counterpart and has potential for use as acceptable human food [23].

According to Aremu et al. [26], *Ganoderma* sp., *Omphalotus olearius*, and *Hebeloma mesophaeum* are species reported to be among the most edible mushrooms commonly found in Nigeria. They evaluated the proximate composition of these three edible mushrooms. The evaluated samples contained moisture, crude protein, ash, crude fat, and total carbohydrate in the range of 10.0–11.1 g/100 g, 18.5–21.5 g/100 g, 7.3–8.3 g/100 g, 6.9–8.7 g/100 g, and 50.3–50.9 g/100 g, respectively. Moreover, Valverde et al. [13] reported that the major fatty acids found in mushrooms are linoleic (C18:2), oleic (C18:1), and palmitic (C16:0). Besides, there was also a mild amount of crude fibre (2.8–3.5 g/100 g) present in the evaluated mushroom [26]. This can be concluded that the nutritional content of mushrooms does not only depend on environmental factors but also on species.

Ishara et al. [30] fortified the maize flour with mushroom flour from *Agaricus bisporus* and *Pleurotus ostreatus*, aimed to improve the nutritional values of the flour. To this, the compositional characteristics and their interactions were investigated. Overall, the protein content of maize flour increased with increased mushroom flour content from 6.9 g/100 g to 15.87 g/100 g (*Agaricus bisporus*) up to 19.32 g/100 g (*Pleurotus ostreatus*), and a significant increase in fibre (*0.53–5.89 g/100 g*) was observed [30]. Overall, edible mushrooms contain a high amount and good quality protein content for approximately 20–40 g/100 g of dry weight basis [31]. They are ranked to be richer than most food sources except meat in terms of protein content [32]. Besides, the mushroom also contains several amino acids that cannot be derived by a human: phenylalanine, lysine, isoleucine, leucine, valine, histidine, threonine, methionine, glutamic acids, and aspartic [5, 33]. To this, glutamic acids and aspartic are the two essential amino acids that give the property umami taste of mushrooms [34]. Therefore, mushroom provides balancing diet compounds in sufficient amounts for human health.

Further, Alexopolous et al. [35] reported that the fairy ring mushroom (*Marasmius oreades*) is a good edible species containing copper, iron, zinc, folic acid, and all the essential amino acids required by a human. In addition, *Lentinula edodes* is reported to have low sodium and glucose, which are ideal for diabetics [35]. In another report, several predominant minerals such as potassium, magnesium, calcium, and iron are found in both exotic cultivated oyster mushrooms and indigenous wild oyster mushrooms. However, most of the mineral values are lower in exotic cultivated mushrooms as compared with that wild oyster mushroom. Oluwafemi et al. [28] reported that phosphorus, magnesium, and potassium were the major abundant minerals in mushroom with 497.35 mg/100 g in the cap, 340.59 mg/100 g stalk, and 466.24 mg/100 g caps with a stalk. Also, according to Kalač [36], potassium is the major element in edible mushrooms. It was reported that potassium is unevenly distributed within the different parts of mushroom fruit bodies; potassium is found to accumulate most concentration in a cap, followed by stipe, spore-forming part, and the least in spores. Magnesium is the second major mineral after potassium found in wild edible mushrooms [36]. Interestingly, sodium is found to present the lowest concentration among all evaluated minerals in the mushrooms [36, 37]. On the other hand, the fortification of maize flour with mushroom powder resulting in the mineral content increased from 2.84 to 8.74 mg/100 g for iron and 3.13 to 5.41 mg/100 g for zinc in the composite flours [30].

Another study was performed on the determination of β-carotene (vitamins A); α-tocopherol and γ-tocopherol for vitamin E, ascorbic acid (vitamin C), thiamine (vitamin B1), and riboflavin (vitamin B2); and several dominant and trace minerals on selected wild edible mushrooms, namely, *Pleurotus* sp., *Hygrocybe* sp., *Hygrophorus* sp., *Schizophyllum commune*, and *Polyporus tenuiculus*. The results revealed that *Schizophyllum commune* had the highest vitamins A and E for approximately 2711.30 mg/g fresh weight and 85.08 mg/g fresh weight, respectively. For other wild edible mushrooms tested, except *Pleurotus* sp., vitamins C, B1, and B2 were found mild [38]. According to Keegan et al. [39], mushrooms generally lacked in vitamin D_2. However, they can act as a biological precursor to vitamin D_2 due to the presence of ergosterol, a type of sterol predominantly found in mushrooms. Therefore, this feature indirectly makes mushrooms as an excellent source for vitamin D_2.

3. Functional properties

The functional properties of flours play an important role in determining the level of utilisation in ingredient formulation as well as in food product development. It is important to recognise the functional properties (i.e. water absorption capacity, oil absorption capacity, emulsifying, foaming, and gelification ability) of mushroom flours for their efficient use and acceptance by consumers [40]. The analysis of functional properties, water absorption capacity, oil absorption capacity, oil emulsion capacity, foaming stability, foaming capacity, least gelation concentration, and bulk density on flour prepared from *Ganoderma* spp., *Omphalotus olearius*, and *Hebeloma mesophaeum* provided interesting findings [26]. The functional properties' results of all the tested edible mushrooms demonstrated that they contained water absorption capacity ranges from 260.0 to 390.0%, 450–480% of oil absorption capacity, 57.3–61.0 mL/g of oil emulsion capacity, foaming stability (51.0–54.0%), foaming capacity ranges from 101.8 to 131.5%, least gelation concentration 12.0–14.0%, and 230.0–410.0 g/mL of bulk density [26]. Moreover, Aremu et al. [26] concluded that the results of forming stability after 24 h for *Ganoderma* spp., *Omphalotus olearius*, and *Hebeloma mesophaeum* reflected that the studied mushroom samples might be attractive for incorporation into meat or bakery products like cakes or whipping topping where oil absorption and foaming are, respectively, important [26]. *Pleurotus sajor-caju* powder presented notable functional properties such as water holding capacity (13.46 g/g), oil holding capacity (8.52 mL/g), swelling capacity (19.49 mL/g), emulsifying activity (51.67%), and emulsifying stability (95.37%) [24].

Cruz-Solorio et al. [29] evaluated the functional properties of flours processed from fruit bodies of three *Pleurotus ostreatus* strains: a strain from commercial (POS), a culture collection strain (PCM) and a hybrid derived from POS and PCM (POS × PCM), and protein concentrates. The authors described pale yellow flours that were obtained from all three strains of edible mushrooms, while greyish brown was observed for protein concentrates. They recorded that the bulk density of the processed flour was to be ranged from 0.52 to 0.64 g/mL which showed higher than that of protein concentrates (0.30–0.35 g/mL). For water absorption capacities, 300–118.8% was obtained for flours, while protein concentrates demonstrated higher oil absorption capacity than the flours. Meanwhile, flours and protein concentrates showed a minimal gelation concentration (2%). For foam capacity formation, protein concentrates presented a higher value than that of flour at pH 8.0. However, for foam stability, both flours and protein concentrates showed high value at pH 8.0 and pH 10.0 (alkaline conditions). The flours presented have 3.96–26.68 m^2/g of emulsion activity index, whereas protein concentrates range from 1.55 to 10.28 m^2/g. The authors concluded that flours and protein concentrates produced from *Pleurotus ostreatus* presented remarkable functional properties and it has the potential to be used in the food industry where foaming and emulsifying properties are required [29].

In addition, another report by Oluwafemi et al. [28] on various parts of *Pleurotus ostreatus* showed that mushroom stalk (675%) had higher water absorption capacity than the cap (487%) and the mixture of stalk and cap (530%). The bulk density varied as 0.483 g/ml cap, 0.297 g/ml stalk, and 0.501 g/ml for a mixture of stalk and cap. Overall, the mushroom cap has the highest emulsion and foaming capacity of 17.33% and 30.67%, respectively. Ishara et al. [30] found that there was a positive significant linear effect in the substitution of mushroom flour (i.e. *Agaricus bisporus* and *Pleurotus ostreatus*) for maize flour on foam stability, foaming capacity, swelling capacity, solubility index, water retention capacity, water absorption capacity, and oil absorption capacity, but a negative linear effect was observed for the bulk density, compact density, and syneresis.

4. Nutraceutical properties

The importance of edible mushrooms as a nutraceutical source can be correlated to their composition and presence of phytochemicals. Reports have shown edible mushrooms to contain a wide array of bioactive compounds. These bioactive compounds present great potential to be applied as therapeutic agents. This is in agreement with the reports from Kozarski et al. [41], whereby the radical scavenging antioxidative activities of edible mushrooms come from an array of biomolecules from the carotenoid and polyphenol groups. Mushrooms are well-known to have rich various bioactive compounds that are widely used as raw material for the development of functional foods. It could emerge as the nutraceutical food for the next generation [42]. According to Sánchez [43], phenolic compounds such as myricetin, quercetin, caffeic acid, catechin, and pyrogallol are present in all edible mushrooms. Besides, antioxidant components (i.e. phenolics, carotenoids, ascorbic acid, tocopherols, ergosterol, and polysaccharides) are mainly found constituted in both fruit bodies, mycelium, and culture of mushrooms [43].

Different edible mushroom cultivars and wild species are reported to possess varied concentrations of phytochemicals and antioxidant activities. Kayode et al. [23] reported that qualitative analysis of oyster mushroom grown on *Gmelina* wood waste and the indigenous wild species of oyster mushroom showed the presence of the five major phytochemicals: alkaloid, tannin, flavonoid, saponin, and cardiac glycosides. In addition, for the quantitative analysis, alkaloid presented as the most predominant phytochemical in both evaluated samples: 10.05% for oyster mushroom grown on *Gmelina* wood waste and 9.64% for indigenous wild species. The authors concluded that oyster mushroom grown on *Gmelina* wood waste could compare favourably with the indigenous wild species counterpart on the phytochemical compositions [23]. Total polyphenols are the dominant naturally occurring antioxidant components found in the wild edible mushrooms that show great scavenging ability due to their hydroxyl groups [44, 45].

Radzki et al. [46] studied the effect of hydrothermal treatment (i.e. citric acid solution blanching (5 min) and oiling in water (15 min)) on the antioxidant capacity (i.e. ferric-reducing antioxidant power assay (FRAP), and scavenging ability on 1,1-diphenyl-2-picrylhydrazyl (DPPH) assays) of three species of edible mushroom, namely, *Pleurotus ostreatus*, *Agaricus bisporus*, and *Lentinula edodes*. The results showed that water extracts for nontreatment mushrooms (control) contained noticeably more phenolic compounds. Both the water and ethanolic extracts for *Agaricus bisporus* possessed the highest content of total phenolic compounds and antioxidant capacity, but the lowest content was found in *Lentinula edodes*. Overall, the authors concluded that the blanching and oiling processes caused a decrease in the antioxidant activity. However, in terms of hydrothermal resistance, *Pleurotus ostreatus* was the most vulnerable [46]. Another report by Mau et al. [47] demonstrated that the methanolic extract of *Termitomyces albuminosus* mycelia has high antioxidant properties. On the other hand, an aqueous extract of *Agaricus blazei* was a potent free radical scavengers and is possible to be used as a pharmacological agent against oxidative stress [48]. Several factors may influence the antioxidant activity of mushroom including the development of fruiting bodies and culture conditions, processing conditions in industrial and domestic environments, and digestion and absorption in human intestinal [49].

Mujić et al. [44] evaluated the potential antioxidant activity content of antioxidant compounds, phenolics and flavonoids, and scavenging capacity on DPPH radicals of three edible mushroom species *Lentinula edodes*, *Hericium erinaceus*, and *Agrocybe aegerita*. *Agrocybe aegerita* showed to have the highest total phenolics (23.07 mg GAE/g) and total flavonoids (5.04 mg CE/g) content. Radical scavenging activity was found to exhibit IC_{50} value for extract concentration of 0.198 mg/mL for *Hericium erinaceus*, 0.073 mg/mL for *Lentinula edodes*, and lower than 0.02 mg/mL for *Agrocybe aegerita*. The highest antioxidant activity of *Agrocybe aegerita* extract is in relation to its highest total phenols content. Therefore, *Agrocybe aegerita* could be considered as a raw material with high potential antioxidant activity [44].

Keleş et al. [45] evaluated total phenolic and antioxidant activity in the methanolic extracts of 24 types of dried wild edible mushrooms. The authors concluded that mushrooms contain 420–12775.56 mg/kg of phenolics and the FRAP and DPPH values range between 145.50–62771.43 μmol/g and 10.17–97.96% of dried matter, respectively; the total phenolics in methanolic extracts were the highest in *Boletus edulis*, whereas the methanolic extracts from *Leccinum scabrum* showed most potent radical scavenging activity (97.96%). It was found that p-coumaric, p-hydroxybenzoic, protocatechuic, and cinnamic acids were contained in the phenolic fraction of five wild mushrooms from Portugal [50]. Thus, edible mushrooms may be applied as natural antioxidants in food products.

5. Therapeutic values

Apart from the nutritional values, edible mushrooms are also being used for a very long time to treat many types of diseases. Many of the common edible species have therapeutic properties and have been eaten for medical treatment purposes [51]. Many therapeutic values of mushrooms traditionally used in folklores of many parts of countries are being scientifically corroborated and have been found to stem from numerous biologically active and health-promoting metabolites that the mushrooms produce [21, 49]. Mushrooms have been reported as useful in preventing diseases such as hypertension, hypercholesterolemia, and cancer [44] due to the presence of high antioxidative compounds in mushrooms. The consumption of food containing antioxidant compounds like mushrooms will protect against the damage of cells from free radical, delays ageing, as well as prevent various diseases [43]. According to Zekovic et al. [52], mushrooms' β-glucans have been reported to exhibit different effects (i.e. antitumour, immune-booster) when compared with β-glucans from oats and barley (i.e. lowering cholesterol and blood sugar). Often, the β-glucans produced by specific mushroom species have specific names such as ganoderan (*Ganoderma lucidum*), grifolan (*Grifola fondosa*), lentinan (*Lentinus edodes*), pleuran (*Pleurotus ostreatus*), and schizophyllan (*Schizophyllum commune*) [53]. Apart from the immunomodulatory properties reported, mushrooms' β-glucans have also been documented to have antibacterial activity [54]. Many studies demonstrated that β-glucans, a water-soluble dietary of many edible mushrooms, are responsible for antioxidant, anticancer, anticholesterolaemic, immunomodulating, and neuroprotective activities. Furthermore, they are recognised as potent immunological stimulators in humans. Studies showed that β-glucans bind to a membrane receptor and induce these biological responses [55–57].

Valverde et al. [13] reported that several active compounds such as phenolics, ascorbic acid, carotenoids, and tocopherol isolated from the different species of mushrooms are responsible compounds to boost the immune system of the body and have anti-hypercholesterolaemic activity, antiviral activity, and anticancer, and ameliorate the toxic effect of chemo- and radiotherapy. The previous study conducted by Lau et al. [58] demonstrated that the protein extract from selected local edible mushrooms (i.e. *Pleurotus cystidiosus* and *Agaricus bisporus*) has high antihypertensive activities. Besides, *Pleuran* from *Pleurotus* spp. has shown marked immunity-stimulating effect and blood cholesterol-reducing effect, whereby proteoglycans possess immunomodulatory and antitumour activities [59]. A similar report was also presented by Li et al. [60]; a polysaccharide isolated from *Pholiota nameko* (PNPS-1) from the family of Strophariaceae leads to significant decreases in very low-density lipoprotein/low-density lipoprotein cholesterol and an increase in high-density lipoprotein cholesterol.

In Japan, lentinan, a complex carbohydrate, is isolated from a variety of mushrooms such as *Lentinula edodes* for the natural treatment of cancer. Lentinan is commonly used in clinic assays as an adjuvant in tumour therapy (i.e. chemotherapy and radiotherapy) [13]. *Lentinula edodes* is also a source of selenium, an antioxidant that is said to prevent cancer [35]. Bioactive proteins and peptides in mushrooms such as lectins, laccases, ribonucleases, antimicrobial proteins, fungal immunomodulatory proteins, and ribosome-inactivating proteins have significant value for pharmaceutical use [61]. According to Zhang et al. [62], lectin isolated from *Pholiota adiposa* showed antiproliferative activity. Lectins are proteins or glycoproteins bound to the carbohydrate cell surface, specifically [63]. Other than that, *Flammulina velutipes* is rich in peroxidase, superoxide dismutase, and others and can prevent some severe diseases like cancer and coronary heart diseases [64]. A study by Qu et al. [65] showed that fatty acids that are extracted from *Hygrophorus eburneus* have antifungal and antibacterial activities. In addition, hygrophamides isolated from the fruiting bodies of *Hygrophorus eburneus* are important constituents of cell membranes that play important roles as antigens and their receptors. Aina et al. [66] recorded that the chanterelles, an edible mushroom species *Cantharellus cibarius*, have antimicrobial activities against yeast, filamentous fungi, Gram-negative and Gram-positive bacteria, as well as actinomycetes.

6. Functional foods from edible mushrooms

Mushrooms are generally traded in food industries in three categories, which are fresh, dried, or canned and processed as mushroom-based products [67]. Most of the fresh mushroom is used in soup, sauce, and as a filling in buns or pizzas. The fresh mushroom is usually sold in local markets due to its short shelf life. As reported by Akbarirad et al. [68], the shelf life of mushrooms is limited under normal refrigeration conditions. The short shelf life of fresh mushrooms is one of the constraints in the distribution and marketing of fresh products. Therefore, in order to maximise the use of mushrooms in the production of high-quality and nutritional food as well as to preserve and ensure that the mushroom can be used for a long period, various mushroom-based products are being developed.

Canned mushrooms have been widely marketed and used in the preparation of mushroom soup, stew, and pizza to replace the use of fresh mushrooms [69–75]. Dried mushrooms have been used in instant soup and sauce preparation [76]. However, the dry form of the edible mushroom has limited uses in food production compared to powdered mushroom which has broad application in food developments. The mushroom powder has great potential as an ingredient in various food products due to its functional characteristics. Mushrooms are recognised as an alternative source of good quality protein and are capable of producing the highest quantity of protein per unit area and time from the worthless agrowastes [77]. Based on a study by Salehi [78], mushrooms contain 22.41% of protein which is higher than the protein in wheat flour. This finding is in line with Wan Rosli et al. [79] and Mendil et al. [80], who reported that the protein content in mushroom is around 25%.

A few studies have been done on supplemented mushroom powdered into food products such as noodles, pasta, rice porridge, as well as bakery products [16, 81–84]. The powder mushroom is mainly being used as a composite flour in bakery production. According to Coelho and Salas Mellado [85], nowadays, there is a lot of attention on the substitution of various flour types for wheat flour to satisfy demands for healthier food. Higher protein content in mushroom powder will develop a better gluten network and produce the right and better elasticity in bakery products as well as in pasta and noodles. The additional amount of mushroom in pasta enhances the antioxidant content [16].

Several studies have been done on the application of mushroom as food additives in food products. Süfer et al. [76] mentioned that the supplemented 5% of *Agaricus bisporus* and *Pleurotus ostreatus* powder in snacks and meatballs gives a promising factor for the production of aromatic and novel foods. The application of mushrooms in meatballs is due to a higher amount of protein and other components such as iron, zinc, selenium, potassium, and vitamin B [86] as well as delicate taste that leads to the growing demand of red meat. Consuming excessive red meat will lead to serious health problems such as cardiovascular diseases, cancer, and obesity due to its saturated fatty acids. The supplemented mushroom powder is expected to reduce the possibility of having those diseases.

7. The effects of edible mushrooms fortification on food quality

The increase in production and consumption of food products using edible mushrooms is due to their nutritional values as well as medicinal effects. Several studies reported that the addition of powdered mushrooms showed an increase in protein, crude fibre, and ash in various food products. Fortification of powdered mushroom at 6 and 10% showed better results for nutritional values as well as the quality for all food products. The protein content in both bread and muffin supplemented with 10% powdered mushroom showed an increase pattern compared to the control. The increase of protein content in both food products was attributed to the high level of protein in mushroom powder. However, the high level of protein content does not affect the specific volume [87]. This suggests that the protein content in powdered mushrooms is unable to produce/develop the gluten network and improve the viscoelasticity of bread and muffin. According to Ortolan and Steel [88], gluten in protein can be categorised into two, which are vital and nonvital glutens. Nonvital gluten is only used for protein enrichment not for its viscoelastic properties.

The crude fibre content in bread is significantly higher than the control [89]. The higher fibre content in food products is favourable due to its beneficial effect on human health such as protection from constipation, cardiovascular diseases, and obesity [90, 91]. The high fibre content in both bakery products is also one of the main reasons for the lower specific volume in bread and muffins. Increasing fibre content in composite flour generally increases the requirement of water absorption [92]. Indirectly it gives heavier loaf and decreases the bread volume. The addition of high fibre content of flour also shows a negative effect on bread quality due to longer dough development, reduction of gas retention, and limitation of expanding the ability of the dough [93].

The supplemented powdered mushroom is high in protein in bakery products such as bread, cake, muffin, and biscuits [81–83, 90]. The addition of 10% of powdered desert truffles may increase the diameter and thickness of the biscuit. According to Gadallah and Ashoush [82], biscuits that have higher spread ratios are considered most desirable. The additional amount of dessert truffle powdered in biscuits is also proven to have higher antioxidant activities.

The enrichment of protein in pasta and noodles can be achieved by adding shiitake, porcini, and powdered oyster mushroom [16, 84]. The moisture content in noodles supplemented with 10% of mushroom powder shows lower enrichment than the control. According to Foschia et al. [94], the reduction of water is due to the competing of fibre in powdered mushrooms with starch during noodle formation, causing the reduction of starch swelling and water absorption. Besides, the fibre content in noodles with 10% additional powdered mushroom shows significant difference with the control which suggests lower moisture content in noodles.

Most of food products such as bread, cake, biscuits, paratha, rice porridge, and noodles show higher ash content compared to control. Higher ash content means a higher amount of mineral present in food products. The taste, texture, appearance, and stability of food products supplemented with powdered mushrooms also depend on the concentration of mineral [81, 82, 90]. The mushroom powder favoured in rice porridge is due to its meaty flavour. Moreover, they contain high protein, fibre, and minerals. The proximate composition and sensory characteristic of rice porridge were investigated by Aishah and Wan Rosli [81]. Their result showed that consumer acceptability of rice porridge supplemented with 6% of oyster mushroom powder has a higher score than the control. A similar trend can be seen in paratha bread [81] except for fat content. Besides, the authors reported that there is a huge reduction of fat content in paratha bread supplemented with 6% of oyster mushroom [81].

Chun et al. [95] used shiitake mushroom in pork patty production. This powdered mushroom acts as phosphate in pork patties. Phosphate acts as food additives, which increase the water holding capacity, reduce cooking loss, and improve the texture of food products. Besides, it also protects the aroma and accelerates the formation of cured meat colour [95]. However, in term of sensory characteristics, most of the food products supplemented with powdered mushrooms were less preferred by the panellists in terms of texture, aroma, taste, and overall acceptability. The colour of food products supplemented with mushroom powder shows darker colour, thus affecting the preference of most mushroom-based products [96].

8. Conclusions

Mushrooms are gaining popularity and are widely consumed across the globe by all age groups. Mushrooms are considered to be one of the superfoods due to its high nutrient content, especially protein, dietary fibre, vitamins, and minerals. In addition, mushrooms are also well-known to contain bioactive compounds, such as ergosterol, β-glucans, lentinan, and peroxidase, which possess health functionalities. This claim is backed by various studies showing that mushrooms possessed anti-hypercholesterolaemic, antiviral, anticancer, and antihypertensive activities. Studies have been conducted to investigate the potential of mushrooms in food applications. The findings from these studies showed promising results, whereby the incorporation of mushroom into food products enhances the nutritional values, as well as the physical properties of the food product. Hence, it is not a surprise to know that the food and pharmaceutical industries are using mushrooms or bioactive compounds from mushrooms to develop functional foods.

Conflict of interest

All authors declare there is no conflict of interest in this review.

Author details

Lee-Hoon Ho[1*], Noroul Asyikeen Zulkifli[1] and Thuan-Chew Tan[2]

1 Faculty of Bioresources and Food Industry, Department of Food Industry, Universiti Sultan Zainal Abidin, Besut, Malaysia

2 Food Technology Division, School of Industrial Technology, Universiti Sains Malaysia, USM, Penang, Malaysia

*Address all correspondence to: holeehoon@yahoo.com; holeehoon@unisza.edu.my

References

[1] Kalaras MD, Beelman RB, Elias RJ. Effects of postharvest pulsed UV light treatment of white button mushrooms (*Agaricus bisporus*) on vitamin D2 content and quality attributes. Journal of Agricultural and Food Chemistry. 2012;**60**:220-225. DOI: 10.1021/jf203825e

[2] Mallikarjuna SE, Ranjini A, Haware DJ, Vijayalakshmi MR, Shashirekha MN, Rajarathnam S. Mineral composition of four edible mushrooms. Journal of Chemistry. 2013;**2013**:1-5. DOI: 10.1155/2013/805284

[3] Feeney MJ, Dwyer J, Hasler-Lewis CM, Milner JA, Noakes M, Rowe S, et al. Mushrooms and health summit proceedings. The Journal of Nutrition. 2014;**144**(1):1128S-1136S. DOI: 10.3945/jn.114.190728

[4] Manjunathan J, Kaviyarasan V. Nutrient composition in wild and cultivated edible mushroom, *Lentinus tuberregium* (Fr.) Tamil Nadu, India. International Food Research Journal. 2011;**18**:809-811

[5] Lallawmsanga, Passari AK, ishra VK, Leo VV, Singh BP, Meyyappan GV, et al. Antimicrobial potential, identification and phylogenetic affiliation of wild mushrooms from two sub-tropical semi-evergreen Indian Forest ecosystems. PLoS One. 2016;**11**(11):e0166368. DOI: 10.1371/journal.pone.0166368

[6] Feng T, Wu Y, Zhang Z, Song S, Zhuang H, Xu Z, et al. Purification, identification, and sensory evaluation of kokumi peptides from *Agaricus bisporus* mushroom. Food. 2019;**8**:1-12. DOI: 10.3390/foods8020043

[7] Ma G, Yang W, Zhao L, Pei F, Fang D, Hu Q. A critical review on the health promoting effects of mushrooms nutraceuticals. Food Science and Human Wellness. 2018;**7**:125-133. DOI: 10.1016/j.fshw.2018.05.002

[8] Cheung LM, Cheung PCK, Ooi VEC. Antioxidant activity and total phenolics of edible mushroom extracts. Food Chemistry. 2003;**81**:249-255. DOI: 10.1016/S0308-8146(02)00419-3

[9] Lallawmsanga, Leo VV, Passari AK, Muniraj IK, Uthandi S, Hashem A, et al. Elevated levels of laccase synthesis by *Pleurotus pulmonarius* BPSM10 and its potential as a dye decolorizing agent. Saudi Journal of Biological Sciences. 2018;**26**(3):464-468. DOI: 10.1016/j.sjbs.2018.10.006

[10] Mishra VK, Passari AK, Leo VV, Singh BP. Molecular diversity and detection of endophytic fungi based on their antimicrobial biosynthetic genes. In: Singh BP, Gupta VK, editors. Molecular Markers in Mycology, Fungal Biology. Switzerland: Springer International Publisher; 2016. pp. 1-35. DOI: 10.1007/978-3-319-34106-4_1

[11] Leo VV, Passari AK, Joshi JB, Mishra VK, Uthandi S, Gupta VK, et al. A novel triculture system (CC3) for simultaneous enzyme production and hydrolysis of common grasses through submerged fermentation. Frontiers in Microbiology. 2016;**7**:447. DOI: 10.3389/fmicb.2016.00447

[12] Kalaras MD, Richie JP, Calcagnotto A, Beelman RB. Mushrooms: A rich source of the antioxidants ergothioneine and glutathione. Food Chemistry. 2017;**233**:429-433. DOI: 10.1016/j.foodchem.2017.04.109

[13] Valverde ME, Hernández-Pérez T, Paredes-López O. dible mushrooms: Improving human health and promoting quality life. International Journal of Microbiology. 2015;**2015**:1-14. DOI: 10.1155/2015/376387

[14] Wan Rosli WI, Solihah MA. Nutritive qualities of patties prepared with mixture of meat and oyster

mushroom. International Food Research Journal. 2014;**21**:2001-2006

[15] Vallée M, Lu X, Narciso JO, Li W, Qin Y, Brennan MA, et al. Physical, predictive glycaemic response and antioxidative properties of black ear mushroom (*Auricularia auricula*) extrudates. Plant Foods for Human Nutrition. 2017;**72**:301-307. DOI: 10.1007/s11130-017-0621-6

[16] Lu XK, Brennan MA, Serventi L, Liu JF, Guan WQ, Brennan CS. Addition of mushroom powder to pasta enhances the antioxidant content and modulates the predictive glycaemic response of pasta. Food Chemistry. 2018;**264**:199-209. DOI: 10.1016/j.foodchem.2018.04.130

[17] Olawuyi IF, Lee WY. Quality and antioxidant properties of functional rice muffins enriched with shiitake mushroom and carrot pomace. International Journal of Food Science and Technology. 2019;**54**:2321-2328. DOI: 10.1111/ijfs.14155

[18] Lu X, Brennan MA, Narciso J, Guan W, Zhang J, Yuan L, et al. Correlations between the phenolic and fibre composition of mushrooms and the glycaemic and textural characteristics of mushroom enriched extruded products. LWT: Food Science and Technology. 2020;**118**:108730. DOI: 10.1016/j.lwt.2019.108730

[19] Royse DJ, Baars J, Tan Q. Current overview of mushroom production in the world. In: Diego CZ, Pardo-Giménez A, editors. Edible and Medicinal Mushrooms: Technology and Applications. West Sussex: John Wiley & Sons Ltd; 2017. pp. 5-13. DOI: 10.1002/9781119149446

[20] FAOSTAT. Mushrooms and Truffles [Internet]. 2019. Available from: http://www.fao.org/faostat/en/#data/QC [Accessed: 12 August 2019]

[21] Samsudin NIP, Abdullah N. Edible mushrooms from Malaysia; a literature review on their nutritional and medicinal properties. International Food Research Journal. 2019;**26**:11-31

[22] Boa E. Wild Edible Fungi—A Global Overview of their Use and Importance to People [Internet]. 2004. Available from: http://www.fao.org/3/y5489e/y5489e00.htm#Contents [Accessed: 12 August 2019]

[23] Kayode RMO, Olakulehin TF, Adedeji BS, Ahmed O, Aliyum TH, Badmos AHA. Evaluation of amino acid and fatty acid profiles of commercially cultivated oyster mushroom (*Pleurotus sajor-caju*) grown on gmelina wood waste. Nigerian Food Journal. 2015;**33**(1):18-21. DOI: 10.1016/j.nifoj.2015.04.001

[24] Han NS, Ahmad WANW, Ishak WRW. Quality characteristics of *Pleurotus sajor-caju* powder: Study on nutritional compositions, functional properties and storage stability. Sains Malaysiana. 2016;**45**(11):1617-1623

[25] USDA. Food Data Central [Internet]. 2019. Available from: https://fdc.nal.usda.gov [Accessed: 12 August 2019]

[26] Aremu MO, Basu SK, Gyar SD, Goyal A, Bhowmik PK, Datta BS. Proximate composition and functional properties of mushroom flours from *Ganoderma* spp., *Omphalotus olearius* (DC.) sing. and *Hebeloma mesophaeum* (Pers.) Quél. used in Nasarawa State, Nigeria. Malaysian Journal of Nutrition. 2009;**15**(2):233-241

[27] Elleuch M, Bedigian D, Roiseux O, Besbes S, Blecker C, Attia H. Dietary fibre and fibre-rich by-products of food processing: Characterisation, technological functionality and commercial applications: A review. Food Chemistry. 2011;**124**:411-421. DOI: 10.1016/j.foodchem.2010.06.077

[28] Oluwafemi GI, Seidu KT, Fagbemi TN. Chemical composition, functional properties and protein fractionation of edible oyster mushroom (*Pleurotus ostreatus*). Annals. Food Science and Technology. 2016;**17**(1):218-223

[29] Cruz-Solorio A, Villanueva-Arce R, Garín-Aguilar ME, Leal-Lara H, Toro GV-D. Functional properties of flours and protein concentrates of 3 strains of the edible mushroom *Pleurotus ostreatus*. Journal of Food Science Technology. 2018;**55**(10):3892-3901. DOI: 10.1007/s13197-018-3312x

[30] Ishara JRM, Sila DN, Kenji GM, Buzera AK. Nutritional and functional properties of mushroom (*Agaricus bisporus* & *Pleurotus ostreatus*) and their blends with maize flour. American Journal of Food Science and Technology. 2018;**6**(1):33-41. DOI: 10.12691/ajfst-6-1-6

[31] Farzana T, Mohajan S. Effect of incorporation of soy flour to wheat flour on nutritional and sensory quality of biscuits fortified with mushroom. Food Science and Nutrition. 2015;**3**(5):363-369. DOI: 10.1002/fsn3.228

[32] Chang ST, Miles PG. Recent trends in world production of cultivated edible mushroom. Mushroom Journal. 1989;**504**:15-17

[33] Wang XM, Zhang J, Wu LH, Zhao YL, Li T, Li JQ, et al. A mini-review of chemical composition and nutritional value of edible wild-grown mushroom from China. Food Chemistry. 2014;**151**:279-285. DOI: 10.1016/j.foodchem.2013.11.062

[34] Tsai SY, Tsai HL, Mau JL. Non-volatile taste components of *Agaricus blazei*, *Agrocybe cylindracea* and *Boletus edulis*. Food Chemistry. 2008;**107**:977-983. DOI: 10.1016/j.foodchem.2007.07.080

[35] Alexopolous CJ, Mims CW, Blackwell M. Introductory Mycology. 4th ed. India: John Wiley & Sons; 2002. pp. 880

[36] Kalač P. A review of chemical composition and nutritional value of wild-growing and cultivated mushrooms. Journal of the Science of Food and Agriculture. 2013;**93**:209-2018. DOI: 10.1002/jsfa.5960

[37] Shin CK, Yee CF, Shya LJ, Atong M. Nutritional properties of some edible wild mushrooms in Sabah. Journal of Applied Sciences. 2007;**7**:2216-2221. DOI: 10.3923/jas.2007.2216.2221

[38] Chye FY, Wong JY, Lee JS. Nutritional quality and antioxidant activity of selected edible wild mushrooms. Food Science and Technology International. 2008;**14**:375-384. DOI: 10.1177/1082013208097445

[39] Keegan RJ, Lu Z, Bogusz JM, Wiliams JE, Holick MF. Photobiology of vitamin D in mushrooms and its bioavailability in humans. Dermato-Endocrinology. 2013;**5**:165-176. DOI: 10.4161/derm.23321

[40] Adebowale K, Lawal O. Comparative study of the functional properties of Bambara groundnut (*Voandzeia subterranean*) jack bean (*Canavalia ensiformis*) and Mucuna bean (*Mucuna pruriens*) flour. Food Research International. 2004;**37**:355-365. DOI: 10.1016/j.foodres.2004.01.009

[41] Kozarski M, Klaus A, Jakovljevic D, Todorovic N, Vunduk J, Petrović P, et al. Antioxidants of edible mushrooms: A review. Molecules. 2015;**20**:19489-19525. DOI: 10.3390/molecules201019489

[42] Rathore H, Prasad S, Sharma S. Mushroom nutraceuticals for improved nutrition and better human health: A review. PharmaNutrition. 2017;**5**:35-46. DOI: 10.1016/j.phanu.2017.02.001

[43] Sánchez C. Reactive oxygen species and antioxidant properties from mushrooms. Synthetic and Systems Biotechnology. 2017;**2**(2017):13-22. DOI: 10.1016/j.synbio.2016.12.001

[44] Mujić I, Zeković Z, Lepojević Ž, Vidović S, Živković J. Antioxidant properties of selected edible mushroom species. Journal of Central European Agriculture. 2010;**11**(4):387-392. DOI: 10.1007/s11483-009-9143-6

[45] Keleş A, Koca I, Gençcelep H. Antioxidant properties of wild edible mushrooms. Food Processing and Technology. 2011;**2**(6):1000130. DOI: 10.4172/2157-7110.1000130

[46] Radzki W, Sławińska A, Jabłońska-Ryś E, Michalak-Majewska M. Effect of blanching and cooking on antioxidant capacity of cultivated edible mushrooms: A comparative study. International Food Research Journal. 2016;**23**(2):599-605

[47] Mau JL, Chang CN, Huang SJ, Chen CC. Antioxidant properties of methanolic extracts from *Grifola frondosa*, *Morchella esculenta* and *Termitomyces albuminosus* mycelia. Food Chemistry. 2004;**87**(1):111-118. DOI: 10.1016/j.foodchem.2003.10.026

[48] Hakime-Silva RA, Vellosa JCR, Khalil NM, Khalil OAK, Brunetti IL, Oliveira OMMF. Chemical enzymatic and cellular antioxidant activity studies of *Agaricus blazei* Murrill. Anais da Academia Brasileira de Ciencias. 2013;**85**(3):1073-1081. DOI: 10.1590/S0001-37652013005000044

[49] Ruiz-Rodriguez A, Santoyo S, Soler-Rivas C. Antioxidant properties of edible mushrooms. Functional Plant Science and Biotechnology. 2009;**3**(Special Issue 1):92-102

[50] Heleno SA, Barros L, Martins A, Queiroz MJRP, Santos-Buelga C, Ferreira ICFR. Portugal: Chemical compounds with antioxidant properties. Journal of Agricultural and Food Chemistry. 2012;**60**(18):4634-4640. DOI: 10.1016/j.foodres.2012.12.020

[51] Guillamón E, García-Lafuente A, Lozano M, D'Arrigo Rostagno MA, Villares A, Martínez JA. Edible mushrooms: Role in the prevention of cardiovascular diseases. Fitoterapia. 2010;**81**(7):715-723. DOI: 10.1016/j.fitote.2010.06.005

[52] Zekovic DB, Kwiatkowski S, Vrvic MM, Jakovljevic D, Moran CA. Natural modified (1→3)-β-glucans in health promotion and disease alleviation. Critical Reviews in Biotechnology. 2005;**25**:205-230. DOI: 10.1080/07388550500376166

[53] Zhu F, Du B, Bian Z, Xu B. β-Glucans from edible and medicinal mushrooms: Characteristics, physicochemical and biological activities. Journal of Food Composition and Analysis. 2015;**41**:165-173. DOI: 10.1016/j.jfca.2015.01.019

[54] Rasmy GE, Botros WA, Kabeil S, Daba AS. Preparation of glucan from *Lentinula edodes* edible mushroom and elucidation of its medicinal value. Australian Journal of Basic and Applied Sciences. 2010;**4**:5717-5726

[55] Ishibashi KI, Miura NN, Adachi Y, Ohno N, Yadomae T. Relationship between solubility of grifolan, a fungal 1,3-β-D-glucan, and production of tumor necrosis factor by macrophages in vitro. Bioscience, Biotechnology and Biochemistry. 2001;**65**(9):1993-2000. DOI: 10.1271/bbb.65.1993

[56] Kataoka K, Muta T, Yamazaki S, Takeshige K. Activation of macrophages by linear (1→3)-β-D-glucans. Implications for the recognition of fungi by innate immunity. Journal of Biological Chemistry. 2002;**227**(39):36825-36831. DOI: 10.1074/jbc.M206756200

[57] Khan MA, Tania M, Liu R, Rahman MM. *Hericium erinaceus*: An edible mushroom with medicinal values. Journal of Complementary and Integrative Medicine. 2013;**10**(1):253-258. DOI: 10.1515/jcim-2013-0001

[58] Lau CC, Abdullah N, Shuib AS, Aminudin N. Proteomic analysis of antihypertensive proteins in edible mushrooms. Journal of Agricultural and Food Chemistry. 2012;**60**:12341-12348. DOI: 10.1021/jf3042159

[59] Agrawal RP, Chopra A, Lavekar GS, Padhi MM, Srikanth N, Ota S, et al. Effect of oyster mushroom on glycemia, lipid profile and quality of life in type 2 diabetic patients. Australian Journal of Medical Herbalism. 2010;**22**(2):50-54

[60] Li H, Zhang M, Ma G. Hypolipidemic effect of the polysaccharide from *Pholiota nameko*. Nutrition. 2010;**26**(5):556-562. DOI: 10.1016/j.nut.2009.06.009

[61] Xu X, Yan H, Chen J, Zhang X. Bioactive proteins from mushrooms. Biotechnology Advances. 2011;**29**(6):667-674. DOI: 10.1016/j.biotechadv.2011.05.003

[62] Zhang GQ, Sun J, Wang HX, Ng TB. A novel lectin with antiproliferative activity from the medicinal mushroom *Pholiota adiposa*. Acta Biochimica Polonica. 2009;**56**(3):415-421. DOI: 10.1155/2014/340467

[63] Singh RS, Bhari R, Kaur HP. Mushroom lectins: Current status and future perspectives. Critical Reviews in Biotechnology. 2010;**30**(2):99-126. DOI: 10.3109/07388550903365048

[64] Sharma VP, Kumar S, Tiwari RP. *Flammulina velutipes*, the Culinary Medicinal Winter Mushroom. Vol. 6. New Delhi: Yugantar Prakashan Pvt. Ltd; 2009. pp. 7

[65] Qu Y, Zhang HB, Liu JK. Isolation and structure of a new ceramide from the Basidiomycete *Hygrophorus eburneus*. Verlag der Zeitchrift für Naturforschung Section B. 2004;**59**:241-244. DOI: 10.1002/(SICI)1099-0690(199801)1998:1<129::AID-EJOC129>3.0.CO;2-A

[66] Aina DA, Jonathan SG, Olawuyi OJ, Ojelabi DO, Durowoju BM. Antioxidant, antimicrobial and phytochemical properties of alcoholic extract of *Cantharellus cibarius*—A Nigerian mushroom. New York Science Journal. 2012;**5**(101):114-120

[67] Mat Amin MZ, Harun A, Wahab MAMA. Status and potential of mushroom industry in Malaysia. Economic and Technology Management Review. 2014;**9b**:103-111

[68] Akbarirad H, Kazemeini SM, Shariaty MA. Deterioration and some of applied preservation techniques for common mushrooms (*Agaricus bisporus* followed by *Lentinus edodes*, *Pleurotus* spp.). The Journal of Microbiology Biotechnology and Food Sciences. 2013;**2**:2398-2402

[69] Cardwell G, Bornman JF, James AP, Black LJ. A review of mushroom as a potential source of dietary vitamin D. Nutrients. 2018;**10**(10):1498. DOI: 10.3390/nu10101498

[70] Dai X, Stanilka JM, Rowe CA, Esteve EA, Nieves C, Spaiser SJ, et al. Consuming *Lentinula edodes* (shiitake) mushrooms daily improves human immunity: A randomized dietary intervention in healthy young adults. Journal of the American College of Nutrition. 2015;**34**(6):478-487. DOI: 10.1080/07315724.2014.950391

[71] Asfors KE, Ley K. Sulfated polysaccharides in inflammation. Journal of Laboratory and Clinical Medicine. 1993;**121**:201-202

[72] Wasser SP. Medicinal mushrooms as a source of antitumor and

immunomodulating polysaccharides. Applied Microbiology and Biotechnology. 2002;**60**:258-274. DOI: 10.1007/s00253-002-1076-7

[73] Tang C, Hoo PC-X, Tan LT-H, Pusparajah P, Khan TM, Lee L-H, et al. Golden needle mushroom: A culinary medicine with evidenced-based biological activities and health promoting properties. Frontiers in Pharmacology. 2016;7:474. DOI: 10.3389/fphar.2016.00474

[74] Alam N, Yoon KN, Lee JS, Cho HJ, Shim MJ, Lee TS. Dietary effect of *Pleurotus eryngii* on biochemical function and histology in hypercholesterolemic rats. Saudi Journal of Biological Sciences. 2011;**18**(4):403-409. DOI: 10.1016/j.sjbs.2011.07.001

[75] Monira S, Haque A, Muhit A, Sarker NC, Alam AHMK, Rahman AA, et al. Antimicrobial, antioxidant and cytotoxic properties of *Hypsizygus tessulatus* cultivated in Bangladesh. Research Journal of Medicinal Plants. 2012;**6**:30-308. DOI: 10.3923/rjmp.2012.300.308

[76] Süfer O, Bozok F, Demir H. Usage of edible mushrooms in various food products. Turkish Journal of Agriculture: Food Science and Technology. 2016;**4**(3):144-149. DOI: 10.24925/turjaf.v4i3.144-149.599

[77] Chandha KL, Sharma SR. Mushroom research in India—History, infrastructure and achievements. In: Chandha KL, editor. Advances in Horticulture. New Delhi: MPH (Malhotra Publishing House); 1995. pp. 1-8

[78] Salehi F. Characterization of different mushrooms powder and its application in bakery products: A review. International Journal of Food Properties. 2019;**22**(1):1375-1385. DOI: 10.1080/10942912.2019.1650765

[79] Wan Rosli WI, Solihah MA, Mohsin SSJ. On the ability of oyster mushroom (*Pleurotus sajor-caju*) conferring changes in proximate composition and sensory evaluation of chicken patty. International Food Research Journal. 2011;**18**(4):1463-1469

[80] Mendil D, Uluozlu OD, Hasdemir E, Caglar A. Determination of trace elements on some wild edible mushroom samples from Kastamonu Turkey. Food Chemistry. 2004;**88**(2):281-285. DOI: 10.1016/j.foodchem.2004.01.039

[81] Aishah MS, Wan Rosli WI. The effect of addition of oyster mushroom (*Pleurotus sajor-caju*) on nutrient composition and sensory acceptation of selected wheat- and rice-based products. International Food Research Journal. 2013;**20**(1):183-188

[82] Gadallah MGE, Ashoush IS. Value addition on nutritional and sensory properties of biscuit using desert truffle (*Terfezia claveryi*) powder. Food and Nutrition Sciences. 2016;**7**:1171-1181. DOI: 10.4236/fns.2016.712109

[83] Farooq M, Rakha A, Ul Hassan J, Fazal R, Saleem M, Saboor M, et al. Physicochemical and nutritional characterization of mushroom powder enriched muffins. International Journal of Fauna and Biological Studies. 2018;5(3):9-16

[84] Wahyono A, Novianti Bakri A, Kasutjianingati. Physicochemical and sensorial characteristics of noodle enriched with oyster mushroom (*Pleurotus ostreatus*) powder. Journal of Physics. Conference Series. 2018;**953**:012120. DOI: 10.1088/1742-6596/953/1/012120

[85] Coelho MS, Salas MM. Effects of substituting chia (*Salvia hispanica* L.) flour or seeds for wheat flour on the quality of the bread. Food Science and Technology. 2015;**60**(2):263-269. DOI: 10.1016/j.lwt.2014.10.033

[86] Wyness L, Weichselbaum E, O'Connor A, Williams EB, Benelam B, Riley H, et al. Red meat in the diet: An update. British Nutrition Foundation Nutrition Bulletin. 2011;**36**:34-77. DOI: 10.1111/j.1467-3010.2010.01871.x

[87] Majeed M, Khan MU, Owaid MN, Khan MR, Shariati MA, Igor P, et al. Development of oyster mushroom powder and its effects on physicochemical and rheological properties of bakery products. Journal of Microbiology, Biotechnology and Food Sciences. 2017;**6**(5):1221-1227. DOI: 10.15414/jmbfs.2017.6.5.1221-1227

[88] Ortolan F, Steel JC. Protein characteristics that affect the quality of vital wheat gluten to be used in baking: A review. Comprehensive Reviews in Food Science and Food Safety. 2017;**16**:369-381. DOI: 10.1111/1541-4337.12259

[89] Okafor J, Okafor G, Ozumba A, Elemo G. Quality characteristics of bread made from wheat and Nigerian oyster mushroom (*pleurotus Plumonarius*) powder. Pakistan Journal of Nutrition. 2012;**11**:5-10. DOI: 10.3923/pjn.2012.5.10

[90] Sivam AS, Sun-Waterhouse D, Quek SY, Perera CO. Properties of bread dough with added fiber polysaccharides and phenolic antioxidants—A review. Journal of Food Science. 2010;**75**(8):163-174. DOI: 10.1111/j.1750-3841.2010.01815.x

[91] Kendall CWC, Esfahani A, Jenkins DJA. The link between dietary fiber and human health. Food Hydrocolloids. 2010;**24**:42-48. DOI: 10.1016/j.foodhyd.2009.08.002

[92] Gajula H. Effect of wheat bran on gluten network formation as studied through dough development, dough rheology and bread microstructure [Thesis]. Kansas: Kansas State University Manhattan; 2017

[93] Sanz Penella JM, Collar C, Haros M. Effect of wheat bran and enzyme addition on dough functional performance and phytic acid levels in bread. Journal of Cereal Science. 2008;**48**:715-721. DOI: 10.1016/j.jcs.2008.03.006

[94] Foschia M, Peressini D, Sensidoni A, Brennan MA, Brennan CS. How combinations of dietary fibres can affect physicochemical characteristics of pasta. Food Science and Technology. 2015;**61**:41-46. DOI: 10.1016/j.lwt.2014.11.010

[95] Chun S, Chambers E, Chambers D. Perception of pork patties with shiitake (*Lentinus edode* P.) mushroom powder and sodium tripolyphosphate as measured by Korean and United States consumers. Journal of Sensory Studies. 2005;**20**:156-166. DOI: 10.1111/j.1745-459X.2005.00016.x

[96] Hourant P. General properties of the alkaline phosphates: Major food and technical applications. Phosphorus Research Bulletin. 2004;**15**:85-94. DOI: 10.3363/prb1992.15.0_85

Chapter 3

Oyster Mushroom Cultivation on Water Hyacinth Biomass: Assessment of Yield Performances, Nutrient, and Toxic Element Contents of Mushrooms

Sunita Bandopadhyay Mukhopadhyay

Abstract

To obtain a cost-effective production of oyster mushrooms, invasive aquatic weed water hyacinth has been tried out as a substrate in different combinations with rice straw (1:1, 1:2, 2:1) for the cultivation of *Pleurotus* species. The yield of mushrooms significantly increases with their 1:1 combination (RS + WH 1:1), especially in the first flush. No significant differences are observed between the nutrient qualities of the oyster mushrooms that grow either on rice straw or on water hyacinth supplemented rice straw (1:1). Minerals (Fe, Cu, Zn) and toxic elements (Pb, Cd, As) though flow from the substrate of RS + WH (1:1) to the mushrooms do not accumulate at a toxic level. The results of the present study indicate that biomass of water hyacinth weed can safely be used with rice straw (1:1) as the alternate substrate for the cultivation of *Pleurotus* species to reduce the cost of production of protein-rich oyster mushroom and to recycle the vast amount of nuisance weed in an eco-friendly way.

Keywords: oyster mushroom cultivation, *Pleurotus florida*, *P. citrinopileatus*, *P. pulmonarius*, aquatic weed, water hyacinth, biological yield, nutrient quality, mineral, toxic elements

1. Introduction

The fruit bodies of the genus *Pleurotus* are generally referred to as 'oyster mushroom.' It is a lignocellulolytic fungus of Basidiomycetes and grows naturally in the temperate and tropical forests [1] on dead and decaying wooden logs, sometimes on dying trunks of deciduous or coniferous woods or decaying organic matter. It is one of the most suitable fungal organisms for producing protein-rich food (mushroom) from various agricultural or forest wastes without composting.

Cultivation of oyster mushroom (*Pleurotus* spp.) has increased greatly throughout the world during last few decades due to the ease of its cultivation on various lignocellulosic wastes, shorter growth time, no need of composting of its substrate, demand for a few environmental control, high yield potential, high nutritional values as well as medicinal values. These features make oyster mushroom cultivation suitable for the beginners and the mushroom farmers with low-tech equipment. The other reason for the great interest in species of *Pleurotus* is that they secrete a wide range of enzymes [2, 3] capable of degrading lignocellulosic biomass. They are therefore capable of growing on a wide range of substrates. Furthermore, some species grow and fruit at a relatively high temperature, a feature that makes for lower production costs in tropical or subtropical areas, or even in temperate regions during the summer season. Due to these advantages of oyster mushroom, many researchers have been striving to make use of different weeds for example, *Typha* sp. [4], *Leonotis* sp., *Sida acuta*, *Parthenium argentatum*, *Ageratum conyzoides*, *Cassia sophera*, *Tephrosia purpurea*, and *Lantana camara* [5, 6] as the substrates for cultivation of *Pleurotus* species with the concept of eradication through utilization [7–9] and cost-effective production of mushroom. The main problem in the cultivation of *Pleurotus* spp. on weed biomass, is their low yield, especially from the second flush. This problem could be overcome by blending weed plants with other commonly used lignocellulosic wastes like rice straw, wheat straw, or sawdust.

Water hyacinth [*Eichhornia crassipes* (Mart.) Solms.], a fast-growing aquatic weed in tropics and sub-tropics causes serious ecological and economic problems by choking water bodies. On the other hand, it has drawn attention as a plant capable of removing toxic heavy metals (e.g., Cr, Cd, Ni, As, Pb, Eu) from wastewater by adsorbing them on its root and is being used in wastewater treatment [8, 10, 11]. Utilization of the vast quantities of this weed available throughout the year, as a low-cost substrate for oyster mushroom cultivation has been reported by several workers [12–14]. But, the information regarding the effect of this weed on the nutritional qualities and the heavy metal bioaccumulation in the harvested oyster mushrooms is not sufficient. Growing up on a substrate contaminated with various toxic elements may cause edible mushrooms to accumulate those elements at higher concentrations [2], as many mushroom species are known to be efficient accumulators of trace elements [15]. Analysis of concentrations of essential mineral elements and non-essential toxic elements (e.g., As, Pb, Cd, Hg) allows the evaluation of the nutritional quality and health risk of food and is thus part of every food safety program. Therefore, as a prerequisite to assess the contribution of these undesirable elements to the dietary intake as per norms of the food safety program, it is worthwhile to evaluate their levels in the mushrooms grown (artificially/naturally) on any substrate and also to report any possible contamination that would represent a health hazard.

Taking stock of the above needs to assess the feasibility of utilizing water hyacinth as a substrate for cost-effective production of oyster mushrooms, the present chapter highlights the study on (i) the biological yields of three species of *Pleurotus* viz., *Pleurotus florida*, *P. citrinopileatus*, and *P. pulmonarius* cultivated separately on different combinations of rice straw and water hyacinth; (ii) the important biochemical and nutrient qualities of the harvested oyster mushrooms; and (iii) the concentrations of mineral elements (Fe, Cu, Zn) and toxic elements (Pb, Cd, As) in the substrate of cultivation as well as in the harvested mushrooms. The study also attempts to assess the contribution of consumption of these oyster mushrooms to the recommended dietary allowances (RDA) or provisional tolerable daily intake set for mineral elements and toxic elements by standard expert council or committee as The National Academies [16], FAO/WHO [17] or Codex Alimentarius [18] of food safety program. The chapter finally summarizes the findings to conclude the feasibility of utilizing the nuisance weed as the low-cost supplement to rice straw for higher yield of oyster mushrooms, which can be consumed safely.

2. Materials and methods

2.1 Cultivation of *Pleurotus* species

2.1.1 Mushroom strains

Three species of *Pleurotus* namely *Pleurotus florida nomen nudum* (Eger), *P. citrinopileatus* Sing., and *P. pulmonarius* (Fr.) Quel., procured from National Center for Mushroom Research and Training (NCMRT), Solan, Himachal Pradesh, India are used for cultivation. The cultures are maintained on Potato-Dextrose-Agar slants and during the period of cultivation, spawns of the mushroom species are prepared with intact wheat grains [19] in autoclavable polypropylene bags (15 × 12 cm).

2.1.2 Substrate

Rice straw (RS) and sun-dried water hyacinth (WH) plants are used as a substrate for the cultivation of *Pleurotus* spp. WH plants are collected locally from the banks of ponds, lakes, and rivers after cleaning of the water bodies. The roots are discarded (as reported to adsorb heavy metals) from the sun-dried plants to use in the preparation of mushroom beds.

2.1.3 Preparation of substrates and cultivation of mushroom

Cultivation trials are conducted at different temperature regimes (different seasons of the year) on five separate combinations of RS and WH (wet weight/wet weight) viz., (i) only RS, (ii) only WH, (iii) RS + WH (1:1), (iv) RS + WH (2:1), and (v) RS + WH (1:2). Both the substrates (RS and WH) are pretreated and the mushroom beds are prepared by packing the substrates in the transparent polythene bags [20]. The beds are then inoculated with 5% (w/w on the wet weight basis) grain spawn of the *Pleurotus* spp. by the layer spawning method [19]. After spawn run (mycelial colonization of the substrate) at 25 ± 2°C and 65 ± 5% relative humidity in the semi-dark condition, fruit body formation is triggered by shifting the environmental variables namely moisture, air exchange, temperature, and light in the cropping room [19]. Fruit primordia (pinhead) are developed within a temperature and relative humidity regimes of 22–30°C and 70–75%, respectively, for the moderate temperature requiring species of *P. citrinopileatus* and *P. pulmonarius*. The low-temperature requiring species of *P. florida* fructify at 14–22°C and 75–80% relative humidity. Mushrooms are harvested manually from each bed when the pinheads are developed to complete fruit body and weighed the same day. The beds are maintained until the harvest of third flush. Production of mushrooms per flush is recorded only at respective optimum temperature regimes (favorable season) of each species to calculate the biological yield per flush [biological yield (B.Y.) = weight of fresh mushrooms harvested (g) per kg dry substrate]. The distribution of the yield (B.Y.) of the experimental species of *Pleurotus* is tabulated to observe any change in the yield over three flushes.

2.2 Nutrient and biochemical qualities of the mushrooms

For proximate analysis of important nutrient and biochemical properties, the mushrooms of each species of *Pleurotus* are harvested from the beds of RS and RS + WH (1:1) separately, oven-dried at 60°C for 72 h and milled to obtain samples of oyster mushrooms (dry weight biomass or DWB). The moisture content of the fresh mushrooms and the total protein (modified Lowry's method), total carbohydrate, vitamins (ascorbic acid and niacin), reducing sugar, crude fiber contents in the DWB are estimated following Sadasivam and Manikam [21]. Exchangeable potassium (by flame photometry method), water-soluble cations (Na^+, K^+, Ca^+) (through ion-exchange chromatography; Metrohm 861 Advanced Compact IC), ash contents, electrical conductivity (EC) and pH in the mushroom samples (DWB) are determined by the methods of Rao and Reddy [22]. Total soluble salt concentration is calculated from EC [21].

2.3 Essential mineral and toxic element contents in the mushrooms and the substrate (RS + WH 1:1) before cultivation

Iron, copper, and zinc (Fe, Cu, Zn), the essential trace elements for human, have been chosen as representative essential minerals and lead, cadmium, arsenic (Pb, Cd, As) as representative toxic elements, whose levels in environment represent a reliable index of environment pollution. Concentrations of these representative minerals and toxic elements in the mushrooms harvested from RS + WH (1:1) beds and in the respective substrates (before cultivation) are determined [23] with atomic absorption spectrometer (AAS) [Perkin Elmer 5100 PC for Cu, Zn, Fe, Pb, and Cd; AVANTA GBC AAS with flamed hollow cathode lamp for As]. Samples of mushroom are prepared by mixing the dry mushrooms of the three species of *Pleurotus* in equal proportions (by weight) and used for AAS estimation after their acid digestion [24]. The concentrations of all the essential mineral and toxic elements are the mean of three replicates and expressed in mg per kg dry weight biomass (mg/kg DWB) of mushroom or substrate.

2.4 Statistical analysis

The experiments on cultivation are laid out in a completely randomized design with five combinations of substrates and three species of *Pleurotus*. All the experiments are performed in triplicates and the data are analyzed using descriptive statistics and also subjected to ANOVA to ascertain any significant difference (at $P \leq 0.05$ for yield and at $P \leq 0.01$ for nutrient qualities) between treatments. Least significant differences (LSD) between the means of biological yields are calculated for the *Pleurotus* spp. [25].

3. Results and discussion

3.1 Yield performances of *Pleurotus* species

Among the three species of *Pleurotus*, *P. citrinopileatus* produces the highest number of fruit bodies per mushroom bed, but the maximum size and weight of the individual fruit body are obtained from *P. florida* (maximum size 22 cm x 17 cm, maximum weight-105 g). Mushroom beds with 1:1 and 1:2 combinations of rice straw and water hyacinth show a faster rate of spawn run, pinhead initiation and earlier harvest of mushroom than other combinations.

Table 1 represents the distribution of the yield (B.Y.) of the three *Pleurotus* species during the period of three flushes on five different combinations of substrates. A perusal of the yield performances (**Table 1**) shows a significant increase in B.Y. of each species on the 1:1 combination of rice straw and water hyacinth (RS + WH 1:1) especially, in the first flush. Although the total yields (g/kg DWB

Substrate combination	Biological yield* (g fresh weight of mushroom/kg dry weight of substrate) of *Pleurotus* spp.								
	Species of oyster (*Pleurotus*) mushroom								
	P. florida			*P. citrinopileatus*			*P. pulmonarius*		
	1st flush	2nd flush	3rd flush	1st flush	2nd flush	3rd flush	1st flush	2nd flush	3rd flush
Rice straw (RS)	581 ± 142	504 ± 84	185 ± 50	617 ± 45	575 ± 21	485 ± 15	558 ± 60	422 ± 46	260 ± 56
Water hyacinth (WH)	606 ± 176	350 ± 14	190 ± 10	607 ± 145	567 ± 15	37 ± 42	624 ± 47	347 ± 10	168 ± 25
RS + WH (1:1)	716** ± 373	489 ± 172	215 ± 111	721** ± 63	505 ± 148	408 ± 226	679** ± 32	522 ± 182	278 ± 30
RS + WH (1:2)	608 ± 270	498 ± 95	232 ± 31	633 ± 10	387 ± 10	18.6 ± 10	608 ± 31	435 ± 33	212 ± 35
RS + WH (2:1)	550 ± 98	540 ± 70	230 ± 28	610 ± 84	514 ± 35	325 ± 21	550 ± 28	340 ± 70	285 ± 50
LSD at 5% level	121.1	79.4	43	60.1	24.6	77	50.3	76.3	39.1

**Results are mean ± standard deviation.*
***Results are significantly different ($P \leq 0.05$) from yields on RS.*

Table 1.
Biological yield of Pleurotus *spp. upto third flush on five combinations of rice straw (RS) and water hyacinth (WH).*

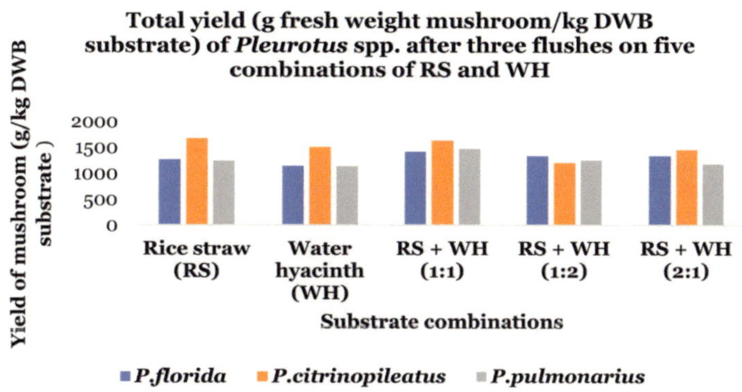

Figure 1.
Total yield of mushrooms (g/kg DWB of substrate) of each of the three species of Pleurotus *after three flushes on each of the five substrate combinations.*

substrate) after three flushes of *P. citrinopileatus* (1634 g/kg), *P. pulmonarius* (1479 g/kg), and *P. florida* (1421 g/kg) (**Figure 1**) on RS + WH (1:1) do not differ significantly. Supplementation of wheat straw with water hyacinth [4] or supplementation of rice straw with different weeds [5] has been reported to increase the yield of mushrooms. Though the negative effect of the weed on the yield of *P. sajor-caju* has also been reported [26]. The better yield with water hyacinth may be due to mitigation of optimal nutritional requirements of mushroom fungi, better aeration and water retention capacity to the mushroom beds by aquatic spongy plant water hyacinth over rice straw up to the stage of fruit body formation. Moreover, supplementation of nitrogen by natural nitrogen-rich supplement as water hyacinth may have resulted in a higher rate of lignocellulolytic degradation. In all the subsequent experiments and analyses of this study, the mushrooms grown on the beds of RS + WH (1:1) are, therefore, taken into consideration for quality assessment.

3.2 Assessment of nutrient quality of mushroom

Comparisons of important nutrient qualities of *Pleurotus* mushrooms harvested from the beds of RS and RS + WH (1:1) reveal no significant differences (**Table 2**) except EC (electrical conductivity). The total protein content of the mushroom varies from 16 to 25% (on the dry weight basis) among the three species of *Pleurotus* (**Table 3**), which are higher than the earlier reports [12] on *P. sajor-caju*. Previous workers have reported protein content ranging from 3 to 5% on the dry weight basis (in *P. florida*, *P. sajor-caju*, and *P. eous*) [27] and from 0.5 to 1% on the fresh weight basis (in *P. ostreatus*) [5] of the oyster mushrooms cultivated on different weeds. The total carbohydrate content of the experimental mushrooms ranges between 19 and 28% (DWB), which is lower than those reported earlier [12, 27]. The vitamin contents of the mushrooms are higher than the earlier reports [12] on *Pleurotus* spp. The crude fiber and the ash contents of the mushrooms are approximately similar to previous findings on *P. sajor-caju* [12]. Electrical conductivity (EC) and as such total soluble salt concentration (calculated from EC) are found to be significantly higher in mushrooms from RS + WH (1:1), which complies with the previous findings [12] in *P. sajor-caju*. The available K^+ content in mushrooms grown on RS +WH (1:1)

Nutrient qualities	Nutritional values* of mushrooms grown on	
	RS	RS + WH (1:1)
Moisture (% FWB)	79.3 ± 11.7	82.7 ± 8.1
Protein (% DWB)	19.2 ± 2.6	22.2 ± 2.7
Carbohydrate (% DWB)	26.5 ± 1.9	22.9 ± 1.7
Vitamins		
(i) Ascorbic acid (% DWB)	0.0133 ± 0.0003	0.0123 ± 0.0002
(ii) Niacin (% DWB)	0.0022 ± 0.0001	0.0013 ± 0.0006
Reducing sugars (% DWB)	3.9 ± 1.3	4.4 ± 1.2
Crude fiber (% DWB)	9.1 ± 0.3	9.4 ± 0.5
Ash (% DWB)	18.5 ± 1.5	18.4 ± 0.7
Exchangeable K^+ (% DWB)	5.1± 0.06	4.4 ± 0.07
Water soluble K^+ (% DWB)	0.13 ± 0.05	0.18 ± 0.06
Water soluble Na^+ (% DWB)	0.04 ± 0.04	0.05 ± 0.04
Water soluble Ca^+ (% DWB)	0.01 ± 0.005	0.01 ± 0.004
EC (electrical conductivity) (mS/cm)	1.5 ± 0.4	2.1 ± 0.2**
pH	6.9 ± 0.3	6.0 ± 0.2

FWB = fresh weight biomass; DWB = dry weight biomass of mushroom.
**Results are mean ± standard deviation.*
***Results are significantly different ($P \leq 0.01$).*

Table 2.
*Comparisons of nutrient and biochemical qualities of oyster mushrooms (*Pleurotus *spp.) grown on rice straw (RS) and water hyacinth supplemented rice straw (RS + WH 1:1).*

Pleurotus spp.	Moisture	Protein	Total soluble salt
	% of fresh weight biomass of mushroom (% FWB)*	% of dry weight biomass of mushroom (% DWB)*	
P. florida	84.9 ± 10	23.8 ± 1.3	0.5 ± 0.7
P. citrinopileatus	81 ± 7	20.8 ± 0.8	0.7 ± 0.5
P. pulmonarius	82 ± 8	16.8 ± 1.3	0.6 ± 0.4

**Results are mean ± standard deviation.*

Table 3.
Moisture, protein and total soluble salt contents of mushrooms of three spp. of Pleurotus *cultivated on RS + WH (1:1).*

exceeds the values in earlier reports [12] for different *Pleurotus* species. But as the recommended dietary allowance (RDA) of potassium is 4.7 g/day/person [16], so these mushrooms (fresh weight) are safe for daily consumption. **Table 3** indicates no significant variation among the experimental mushroom species (*P. florida*, *P. citrinopileatus*, and *P. pulmonarius*) in their moisture, total protein and, total soluble salt contents.

3.3 Assessment of mushroom quality based on the levels of important mineral and toxic elements

Table 4 depicts the concentrations (mg/kg DWB) of representative essential minerals (Fe, Zn, and Cu) and non-essential toxic metals (Pb, Cd, and As) in the harvested mushrooms as well as in their respective substrates (RS + WH 1:1) before cultivation. The results are consistent with the previous studies on cultivated mushrooms and except arsenic [24], fall within the range reported for *Pleurotus* mushrooms in the literature [24, 28–31].

Mineral/toxic element	Concentration** (mg/kg DWB* of substrate) of mineral and toxic element in the substrate (RS + WH 1:1) before cultivation	Concentration** (mg/kg DWB* of mushroom) of mineral and toxic element in the mushrooms of the present study	Range of mineral and toxic element contents in cultivated spp. of *Pleurotus* in published literature (mg/kg DWB* of mushroom)	References
Iron (Fe)	295 ± 104.3	216 ± 92.3	67–1524	[24, 28–30]
Zinc (Zn)	56.5 ± 6.2	53.1 ± 5	54–180	[28–30]
Copper (Cu)	11.9 ± 2.6	12.1 ± 0.9	11–182	[28–30]
Lead (Pb)	7.2 ± 1.2	2.2 ± 1.1	n.d.–4.4	[28, 29, 31]
Cadmium (Cd)	2.7 ± 1.8	1.8 ± 0.8	0.3–2.9	[24, 28–30]
Arsenic (As)	3.4 ± 0.06	0.5 ± 0.3	0.04	[24]

**DWB = dry weight biomass.*
***Results are mean ± SD.*

Table 4.
Concentrations (mg/kg) of minerals and toxic elements in the mushrooms and respective substrate before cultivation (RS + WH 1:1) in the present study and the range of their concentrations in selective references.

3.3.1 Bioaccumulation factor

The bioaccumulation factor represents the element concentration in mushrooms compared with its concentration in the environment (in soil/substrate) [32]. The ability of mushrooms to accumulate elements from the substrates [15] is expressed by a bioaccumulation factor or co-efficient of accumulation (K_a), which is the ratio of the concentration (on the dry weight basis) of an element in the mushrooms (C_m) to the concentration (on the dry weight basis) in the underlying substrate (C_s) ($K_a = C_m/Cs$). K_a of the representative elements in the studied mushrooms are presented in **Table 5**, which shows the bioaccumulation factor in the descending order of Cu > Zn > Fe > Cd > Pb > As. This indicates higher mobility of copper than the zinc or iron in the analyzed species of mushrooms. Lead and arsenic are accumulated at minimal levels. The bioaccumulation factor for lead decreases as its concentrations in substrate increases. Thus, the studied oyster mushroom has probably a regulative mechanism for lead intake. Similar findings have been reported in the literature for cadmium uptake in *Pleurotus ostreatus* [15]. Levels of the undesirable metals are considerably lower in the cultivated mushrooms than in the same or taxonomically-related wild-growing species [15]. For a plant or mushroom to be efficient bio-accumulator, the bioaccumulation factor has to be higher than one [32]. Therefore, it is obvious that in the present study although the toxic elements are present in the initial substrates of cultivation (water hyacinth supplemented rice straw 1:1), but are not accumulating at toxic levels in the mushrooms.

3.3.2 Contribution of the mushroom consumption to the dietary intake

In order to contribute to the safe consumption of the experimental mushrooms (grown on RS + WH 1:1) to the dietary intake of essential minerals and to evaluate the risk of dietary exposure to the toxic elements, the concentrations of the representative elements are compared with the recommended values of dietary intake for an average adult of 60 kg body weight (b.w.) set by standard international organizations [16–18]. As the recommended values are based on the fresh weight of mushroom, the mineral and toxic element contents (on the dry weight basis) are converted on the scale for 100 g fresh mushroom (considering 82 % average moisture content of the experimental mushrooms) and presented in **Table 6**. The concentrations of Fe, Zn, Cu, Pb, Cd, and As are found to be approximately

Mineral/toxic element	Concentration of mineral/ toxic element (mg) in the mushrooms produced per kg DWB of substrate (considering 82% moisture content of the mushrooms) (C_m)	Concentration of mineral and toxic element (mg) per kg DWB of substrate (rice straw + water hyacinth 1:1) (C_s)	Bioaccumulation factor or coefficient of accumulation ($K_a = C_m/C_s$)
Iron (Fe)	61.6	295	0.21
Zinc (Zn)	15.1	56.5	0.26
Copper (Cu)	3.4	11.9	0.28
Lead (Pb)	0.62	7.2	0.09
Cadmium (Cd)	0.51	2.7	0.19
Arsenic (As)	0.14	3.4	0.04

Table 5.
Bioaccumulation factor (K_a) of the mineral and toxic elements in the mushrooms produced on RS + WH (1:1).

Mineral/toxic element	Recommended values of dietary intake (derived from RDA[*,a,b]/PTWI[**,c]) mg/day/person	Mineral/toxic element content (mg) per 100 g fresh weight of experimental mushroom
Iron (Fe)	8/18 (male/female)[a]	3.8
Zinc (Zn)	11/8 (male/female)[a]	0.95
Copper (Cu)	0.9[a]	0.21
Lead (Pb)	0.2[b]	0.04
Cadmium (Cd)	0.06[b]	0.03
Arsenic (As)	0.12–0.42[c]	0.009

[*]RDA, recommended dietary allowances.
[**]PTWI, provisional tolerable weekly intake.
[a]Referred to National Research Academies, 2006 [16].
[b]Codex Alimentarius, 2011 [18].
[c]Joint FAO/WHO expert committee, 2010 [17].

Table 6.
Recommended dietary intake (mg/day/person).[*]

equivalent to 3.8, 0.95, 0.21, 0.04, 0.03, and 0.009 mg, respectively, per 100 g fresh mushroom. Recommended dietary allowances (mg/day) of iron, zinc, and copper for average adult persons are 8/18, 11/8 (male/female), and 0.9, respectively [16], while provisional tolerable daily intake (PTDI) for Cd and Pb are 0.2 and 0.06, respectively [18]. Commission Regulation (EC) [33] has set maximum levels of Cd and Pb at 0.2 mg/kg wet weight and 0.3 mg/kg wet weight, respectively in oyster mushrooms like *Pleurotus ostreatus* [33]. For arsenic, the safe range value in toxicological guidance is 2–7 μg/kg body weight per day [17] allowing 0.12 mg of arsenic to be consumed daily by a person of 60 kg in weight. Considering the above-recommended values, an adult person can, therefore, safely consume 100 g of these experimental mushrooms daily without exceeding (**Table 6**) the permissible levels set by standard expert committee or commission for human consumption.

4. Conclusion

The above study indicates that the supplementation of rice straw with the weed water hyacinth supports a higher yield of oyster mushrooms and also reduces the production time of mushrooms. The small-scale mushroom farms or enterprises can maintain consistency in the supply of mushrooms throughout the year by cultivating different species of *Pleurotus* at their optimum temperatures in the same cropping room. The nutrient qualities of the mushrooms grown on common substrate rice straw are not adversely affected by the supplementation with water hyacinth. Besides, these oyster mushrooms will serve as good sources of protein as well as iron, zinc, and copper. The undesirable elements like lead, cadmium, or arsenic although translocated from the substrate to the mushroom, are not accumulating therein and their levels in the mushrooms fall in line with the recommendations by standard expert committee or commission. Regarding heavy metal contamination, the presence of some heavy metals in soil, air, water, and living objects are unavoidable contaminants and regular monitoring of these toxic elements in the mushrooms grown naturally or artificially is required to do vegetable safety. Utilization of water hyacinth as an alternate substrate for oyster mushroom cultivation can therefore contribute to reducing the cost of mushroom production as well as alleviating its adverse ecological impact. This will change the status of the aquatic weed from prolific pest to the potential provider of protein-rich mushroom, whose controlled consumption daily will not pose any toxicological risk.

Acknowledgements

The author sincerely thanks the Department of Science and Technology, New Delhi, Govt. of India for providing financial assistance under the "Women Scientists Scholarship Scheme for Societal Programmes".

Author details

Sunita Bandopadhyay Mukhopadhyay
Department of Botany, Sonamukhi College, Sonamukhi, Bankura, W.B., India

*Address all correspondence to: sunita_babli@rediffmail.com

References

[1] Lallawmsanga, Passari AK, Mishra VK, Leo VV, Singh BP, Meyyappan GV, et al. Antimicrobial potential, identification and phylogenetic affiliation of wild mushrooms from two sub-tropical semi-evergreen indian forest ecosystems. PLoS ONE. 2016;**11**(11):e0166368

[2] Lallawmsanga, Leo VV, Passari AK, Muniraj IK, Uthandi S, Hashem A, et al. Elevated levels of laccase synthesis by *Pleurotus pulmonarius* BPSM10 and its potential as a dye decolorizing agent. Saudi Journal of Biological Sciences. 2018;**26**(3):464-468

[3] Mishra VK, Passari AK, Leo VV, Singh BP. Molecular diversity and detection of endophytic fungi based on their antimicrobial biosynthetic genes. In: Singh BP, Gupta VK, editors. Molecular Markers in Mycology, Fungal Biology. Switzerland: Springer International Publisher; 2016. pp. 1-35

[4] Mshandete AM. Cultivation of *Pleurotus* HK-37 and *Pleurotus sapidus* (oyster mushrooms) on cattail weed (*Typha domingesis*) substrate in Tanzania. International Journal of Research in Biological Sciences. 2011;**1**:35-44

[5] Das N, Mukherjee M. Cultivation of *Pleurotus ostreatus* on weed plants. Bioresource Technology. 2007;**98**(14):2723-2726. DOI: 10.1016/j.biortech.2006.09.061

[6] Mintesnot B, Ayalew A, Kebede A. Evaluation of biomass of some invasive weed species as substrate for oyster mushroom (*Pleurotus* spp.) cultivation. Pakistan Journal of Biological Sciences. 2014;**17**(2):213-219. DOI: 10.3923/pjbs.2014.213.219

[7] Sharma A. Eradication and utilization of water hyacinth—A review. Current Science. 1971;**40**(3):51-55

[8] Gopal S: Researchers Innovate to Make Money Out of Water Hyacinth. 2018. Available from: https://india.mongabay.com

[9] Leo VV, Passari AK, Joshi JB, Mishra VK, Uthandi S, Gupta VK, et al. A novel triculture system (CC3) for simultaneous enzyme production and hydrolysis of common grasses through submerged fermentation. Frontiers in Microbiology. 2016;**7**:447

[10] Dos Santos MC, Lenz E. The use of aquatic macrophytes (*Eichhornia crassipes*) as a biological filter in the treatment of lead contaminated effluents. Environmental Technology. 2000;**21**:615-622

[11] Aboul-Enein AM, Al-Abd AM, Shalaby EA, Abul-Ela F, Nasr Allah AA, Ahmoud AM, et al. *Eichhornia crassipes* (Mart.) Solms: From water parasite to potential medicinal remedy. Plant Signalling and Behavior. 2011;**6**:834-836

[12] Anakalo Kihumbu G, Shitandi AA, Mahungu MS, Khare KB, Sharma HK. Nutritional composition of *Pleurotus sajor-caju* grown on water hyacinth, wheat straw, and corncob substrates. Research Journal of Agriculture and Biological Sciences. 2008;**4**:321-326

[13] Bandopadhyay Mukhopadhyay S, Chatterjee NC. Water hyacinth, a low-cost supplement for oyster mushroom (*Pleurotus florida*) cultivation. Mushroom Research. 2009;**18**(1):5-9

[14] Singh BP, Chhakchhuak L, Passari AK, editors. Biology of Macrofungi. Switzerland: Springer International Publisher; 2018. DOI: 10.1007/978-3-030-02622-6

[15] Kalac P, Svoboda L. A review of trace element concentrations in edible mushrooms. Food Chemistry. 2000;**69**:273-281

[16] Otten JJ, Hellwig JP, Meyers LD. Dietary Reference Intakes: The Essential Guide to Nutrient Requirements. Washington, D.C.: The National Academies Press; 2006. pp. 1-1344. ISBN: 0-309-10091-7. Available from: http://www.nap.edu/catalog/11537.html

[17] Joint FAO/WHO Expert Committee on Food Additives. Seventy-third Meeting. 8-17 June 2010; Summery and Conclusions. Issued 24th June 2010; Geneva. Available from: http://www.fao.org/ag/agn/jecfa/jecfa73sc.pdf

[18] Codex Alimentarius. Joint FAO/WHO Food Standards Programme Codex Committee on Contaminants in Foods. Fifth Session. CF/5 INF/1. 21-25 March 2011; The Hague. The Netherlands; 2011

[19] Suman BC, Sharma VP. Steps in Mushroom Growing: Mushroom Cultivation and Uses. Jodhpur, India: Agrobios; 2007. pp. 70-270. ISBN: 81-7754-248-6

[20] Bandopadhyay S. Effect of supplementing rice straw with water hyacinth on yield and nutritional qualities of oyster mushroom (*Pleurotus* spp.). Micologia Aplicada International. 2013;**25**(2):15-21

[21] Sadasivam S, Manickam A. Biochemical Methods. 2nd ed. Tamilnadu Agricultural University: New Age International (P) Limited; 1996. pp. 6-12

[22] Rao AS, Reddy KS. Analysis of soils for pH, EC and available major nutrients. In: Tandon HLS, editor. Methods of Analysis of Soils, Plants, Waters, Fertilizers and Organic Manures. New Delhi: Fertilizer Development and Consultation Organisation; 2005. pp. 23-27

[23] Helrich K, editor. Official Methods of Analysis of Association of the Official Analytical Chemists. Agricultural chemicals; Contaminants; Drugs; Vol. 1. 15th ed. Virginia 22201 USA: Association of Official Analytical Chemists, Inc.; 1990. p. 1213. ISBN: 0-995584-42; ISSN: 006696IX

[24] Quarcoo A, Adotey G. Determination of heavy metals in *Pleurotus ostreatus* (Oyster mushroom) and *Termitomyces clypeatus* (Termite mushroom) sold on selected markets in Accra, Ghana. Mycosphere. 2013;**4**(5):960-967

[25] William LJ, Abdi H. Fisher's least significant difference (LSD) test. In: Salkind N, editor. Encyclopedia of Research Design. Sage, Thousand Oaks: CA; 2010. DOI: 10.4135/9781412961288.n154

[26] Shah F, Khan SS, Khan M, Tanveer A. Cultivation of *Pleurotus sajor-caju* on wheat straw, water hyacinth and their combinations. Indian Journal of Fundamental and Applied Life Sciences. 2011;**1**:56-59

[27] Naraian R, Dixit B. Nutritional value of three different oyster mushrooms grown on cattail weed substrate. Archives of Biotechnology and Biomedicine. 2017;**1**:061-066

[28] Akyuz M, Kirbag S. Element contents of *Pleurotus eryngii* (DC. ex Fr.) Quel. var. *eryngi*i grown on some various agro-wastes. Ekoloji. 2010;**19**(74):10-14

[29] Gebrelibanos M, Megersa N, Taddesse AM. Levels of essential and non-essential metals in edible mushrooms cultivated in Haramaya, Ethiopia. International Journal of Food Contamination. 2016;**3**:2. DOI: 10.1186/s40550-016-0025-7

[30] Dogan HH, Sanda MA, Uyanoz R, Ozturk C, Çetin U. Contents of metals in some wild mushrooms: Its impact in human health. Biological Trace Element Research. 2006;**110**:79-94

[31] García MÁ, Alonso J, Melgar MJ. Lead in edible mushrooms: Levels and bioaccumulation factors. Journal of Hazardous Materials. 2009;**167**:777-783

[32] Scragg A. Environmental Biotechnology. 2nd ed. New York: Oxford University Press; 2005. ISBN-10:0199268673; ISBN-13:9780199268672

[33] Commission Regulation (EC) No 1881/2006 of 19 December 2006 setting maximum levels for certain contaminants in foodstuffs. Official Journal of the European Union. 20.12.2006; OJL 364. pp. 5-24

Chapter 4

Mushroom Polysaccharides: Chemistry and Anticancer Potentials

Moyen Uddin Pk, Rumana Pervin, Jabin Jahan, Rabiul Islam Talukder, Sourav Ahmed and Matiar Rahman

Abstract

Mushrooms have been used as a common folk medicine due to their effective bioactive compounds including polysaccharides. It is known that the glucans are the main bioactive mushroom polysaccharides. This review study explains the method of isolation, structural characterization, and antitumor activities of mushroom polysaccharides. In many laboratories, these trials are still underway, and the function of polysaccharides as an antitumor agent is particularly under intense discussion. This review aims to summarize the accessible data and reflect this study area's current status with a perspective to future direction.

Keywords: polysaccharides, edible mushrooms, immunomodulation, glucans, tumoricidal

1. Introduction

Polysaccharides obtained from mushrooms have played a significant role as food and medicinal agent in the therapy of cancer in Asian nations such as China and Japan [1]. The consumption of fresh or dried mushroom powder in pre- and postmenopausal females might prevent breast cancer [2]. Mushrooms with distinctive fruiting bodies that have an impact on cancer curing belong to *Basidiomycetes* class and sometimes *Ascomycetes* classes. The main typical taxa are *Ganoderma lucidum*, *Lentinus edodes*, *Tremella fuciformis*, and *Pleurotus ostreatus*. For the first time in 1957, Lucas verified the bioactivity of *Basidiomycetes* mushrooms. Lucas isolated a *Boletus edulis* substance with an important inhibitory impact on tumor cells from sarcoma S-180 [2]. In 1966, Gregory conducted an extensive study, using submerged fermentation to the respective mushroom types, to isolate the active substances from fruiting bodies of mushroom species [3]. Applied to rodent animal model antitumor testing for the active agents, polysaccharides, which were isolated from 22 mushroom species, had inhibitory effects on tumor cells like sarcoma S-180, adenocarcinoma 755, and leukemia L-1210 [4].

2. Chemistry of polysaccharides

Polysaccharides are the most recognized and powerful mushroom-derived substances with antitumor and immunomodulating characteristics. Because of its wide biological range, polysaccharide β-glucan is the most versatile metabolite. The β-glucans consist of a backbone of glucose residue associated with β-(1 to 3) glycosidic bonds, often connected by β-(1 to 6) linkages with the adjoining side-chain glucose residue [5]. It may be linear or branched to polysaccharides. Polysaccharides are split into two groups according to the number of distinct monomers: homopolysaccharides consist of only one type of monosaccharides, whereas heteropolysaccharides consists of two more types of monosaccharides [6]. Homopolysaccharides and heteropolysaccharides may have homolinkages or heterolinkages in configuration and/or position of connection. Polysaccharides with a powerful antitumor action vary significantly in their chemical structure. Antitumor activity is shown by a broad spectrum of glycans ranging from homopolymers to extremely complicated heteropolymers [7]. A broad variety of antitumor or immunostimulating polysaccharides were explored from distinct chemical structures from greater *Basidiomycetes* mushrooms, and the primary kinds are listed in **Table 1**.

Antitumor polysaccharides comprise monosaccharides like glucose, mannose, xylose, fucose, arabinose, galactose, glucuronic acid, and ribose. In few mushrooms, polysaccharides are conjugated with peptides or proteins which exhibited potent anticancer activity [8]. The origin, type, and bioactivity of the most common edible mushrooms, in Bangladesh, are given in **Table 2**. Some of them have been sold for clinical treatment in patients receiving anticancer treatment with polysaccharides and polysaccharide conjugates.

Glycans are structurally diversified. There are no unique protocols for the analysis of glycans. The primary structure of mushroom polysaccharide comprises the sequence and composition of monosaccharide, position, and configuration of monosaccharide, nature, and number of noncarbohydrate moieties.

During structure analysis, the composition of monosaccharide gives information on the molar ratio of monomers and nature and the location of glycosidic linkages,

Polysaccharides	Glycosidic linkage
Linear	
Amylose	α-(1 → 4)-Glc
Xylan	β-(1 → 4)-Xyl
β-Glucan	β-(1 → 4, 1 → 3)-Glc
Branched	
Amylopectin	α-(1 → 4, 1 → 6)-Glc
Glycogen	α-(1 → 4, 1 → 6)-Glc

Table 1.
Examples of homopolysaccharides [8].

Mushrooms	Polysaccharide source	Type	Bioactivity
Ganoderma lucidum [9]	Fruiting bodies	Heteroglycan Glycopeptide	Antitumor Antioxidative Immunomodulating
Lentinus edodes [10]	Fruiting bodies	Glucan	Antitumor Immunomodulating
Pleurotus tuber-regium [11]	Fruiting bodies Mycelium	B-D-glucan	Anticancer Hepatoprotective

Table 2.
Common edible mushrooms in Bangladesh.

Methods	Structural features
GLC-FID, GLC-MS, HPLC	Monosaccharide compositions
IR, NMR	Glycosidic bonds, configuration
NMR	Sequence analysis

Table 3.
Common methods for primary structure analysis of polysaccharide [12].

detection, and quantification of monomers. In **Table 3**, we represented the analytical methods that are used to analyze the primary structures of polysaccharides.

3. Purification of polysaccharides

Mushroom polysaccharide consists of two main polysaccharide kinds as the structural elements of the fungal cell wall. The celluloses and matrix-like glycoprotein are a rigid cellulose fibrilla, α-glucan or β-glucan. The selection of mushroom polysaccharides is usually based on the cell wall structure. A reliable procedure has been developed for successful polysaccharide mining of either cultivar mycelia or fruit body [13]. The process of extraction usually involves 80% ethanol to remove low molecular substances from the pest material and 3–5 repeated water extractions (100°C, 2–4 h). Alternatively, 5% sodium hydroxide (80°C, 6 h) or 2% ammonium oxalate (100°C, 6 h) is used. Using a mixture of methods such as ethanol precipitation, fractional precipitation, acidic precipitation with acetic acid, ion-exchange chromatography, gel filtration, and chromatography of affinity, extracted polysaccharides can be further purified. The precipitation of ethanol excludes polysaccharides from the impurities. Acidic and neutral polysaccharides can be separated on a DEAE-cellulose column by anion-exchange chromatography. First, a suitable running buffer elucidates the neutral polysaccharide in the blend; then the acid polysaccharide is eluted at a greater salt concentration [14]. Using gel filtration and affinity chromatography, neutral polysaccharides can be further divided into α-glucans (adsorbed fraction) and β-glucans (non-adsorbed fraction). Affinity chromatography is a selective adsorption method and the subsequent regeneration from an immobilized ligand of a compound. This method now enables some carbohydrates to be extremely specific and efficiently purified [15]. Previous studies have indicated that the mushroom sample fractionation for polysaccharides usually began with the extraction of warm water. Pk et al. described the isolation and characterization and anticancer effect of antioxidant polysaccharide from *Pleurotus ostreatus* [16].

4. Anticancer role

4.1 *Pleurotus ostreatus*

Pleurotus ostreatus protein extracts demonstrated therapeutic effectiveness against human colorectal adenocarcinoma cells and cells of human monocytic leukemia [17]. Cao et al. investigated that the colony-forming potential of the BGC-823 cells was significantly reduced, after *Pleurotus ostreatus* polytherapy [18]. Ivette González-Palma et al. (2016) studied the antioxidant properties of fungi *Pleurotus ostreatus* obtained from a local farm in Thailand [19]. Studies of histopathology confirmed the hepatoprotective effect of *P. ostreatus* extract. Such findings suggest that a *P. ostreatus* extract can significantly reduce hepatotoxicity [20]. Vamanu isolated exopolysaccharides and internal polysaccharides from *Pleurotus ostreatus* and investigated in vitro antioxidant activity revealed strong antioxidant ability, which was demonstrated by the EC50 value for DPPH, ABTS scavenging activity, energy reduction, and iron-chelating operation [21]. **Figure 1** shows the concentration effects of polysaccharides from *Pleurotus ostreatus*.

The antimicrobial activity of *P. ostreatus* extracts was determined by the disc diffusion method for Gram-negative bacteria and Gram-positive bacteria. The acetone extracts had antimicrobial activity against only *B. subtilis* and *E. coli*, while the other extracts inhibited the growth of most oral bacteria, indicating a significant growth inhibition of *S. sanguinis* [22].

4.2 *Ganoderma lucidum*

G. lucidum polysaccharides perform anticancer action, by inhibiting the development and growth of the tumors [23], by increasing the immune function of patients, and by different mechanisms, such as anti-proliferating, anti-metastatic [24], antioxidant, and immunomodular [25] (**Figure 2**).

GLP shows activity against cancer by inducing immune responses and directly cytotoxic effects on tumor cells. GLP blocked the proliferation of mouse melanoma cells (B16F10) and human bladder cancer cells (HUC-PC and MTC-11). Several studies have found the mechanism of GLP anticancer role [26].

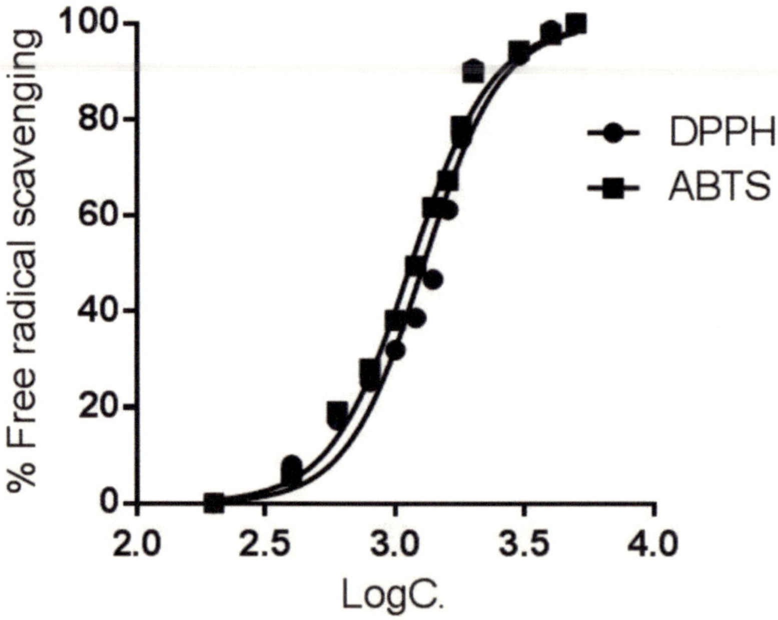

Figure 1.
The effects of POP on DPPH and ABTS radical scavenging.

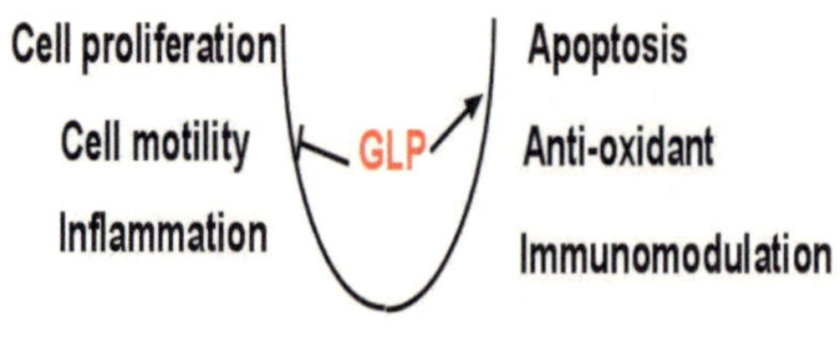

Figure 2.
Ganoderma lucidum *polysaccharides (GLP) results associated with cancer. Arrows are activation, but bars are inhibition.*

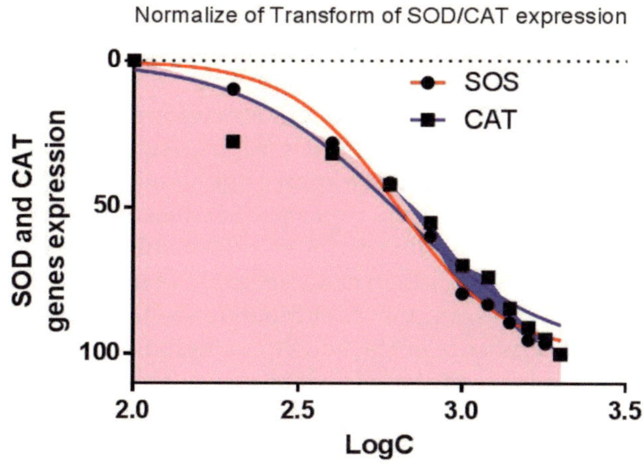

Figure 3.
Tentative relationship between SOD and CAT expressions and Ganoderma lucidum.

Mechanism 1: GLP downregulation of cyclin D1 in human ovarian OVCAR-3 cells is associated with growth inhibition and cell cycle arrest [27].

Mechanism 2: The anticancer activity of GLP includes both phosphoinositide 3-kinase (PI3K)/AKT/mammalian rapamycin (mTOR) and MAPK signaling pathways [28].

Mechanism 3: GLP decreases the expression of certain signaling molecules at gene and protein levels in the PI3K/AKT/mTOR and MAPK pathways [29].

It has been shown that many plants contain high levels of natural antioxidants that can scavenge free radicals [30]. In addition, this property may well decrease the level of DNA damage caused by oxidative stress and thus partially account for chemopreventive mechanisms that are attributed to antioxidants derived from plants [31]. Both the extracts of triterpene and polysaccharide have an antioxidant effect on pyrogallol-induced membrane oxidation and lipid peroxidation mediated by Fe(II)-ascorbic acid [32]. The findings of this study showed that GL extracts displayed dose-dependent antioxidant activity by increasing the expression of SOD and catalase [33]. **Figure 3** shows the expression patterns of SOD and CAT genes.

4.3 *Lentinus edodes*

As edible and medicinal tools, *Lentinus edodes* are appreciated. The most active antitumor and immunomodulatory agents in *Lentinus edodes* have been found to be polysaccharides. Lentinan is an isolated component of highly distilled polysaccharide from *Lentinus edodes* (shiitake). It is known as a β-glucan in terms of its chemical composition. The main chain consists of glucose units bound by β-(1–3) glycosidic bonds, while β-(1–6) glycosidic bonds link side chains with the main chain [13]. It is an authorized anticancer drug that is widely used in Japan. It is commonly used in cancer therapy in combination with other traditional pharmaceutical drugs, e.g., against cancer of the bowel, liver, stomach, ovary, and lung. It increases the efficacy of treatment and therefore the survival of patients [34].

5. Chemical structure

The chemical structure of lentinan has a main chain consisting of β-D-(1 → 3)-linked D-glucopyranosyl residues with two (1 → 6)-β-glucoside branches for every five D-glucose residues, and the side chains of lentinan consist of β-D-(1,6)-linked and β-D-(1 → 3)-linked glucose residues [35] (**Figure 4**).

It has been shown that many mushroom β-glucans stimulate production of interferons (IFNs), interleukins (ILs), and other cytokines [34]. It is based mainly on the activation of T and B lymphocytes, macrophages, and natural killer cells [36]. Studies have found that the proliferation of mononuclear blood cells including lymphocytes, monocytes, and macrophages is induced by lentinan [37]. In addition, the production and differentiation of cells involved in the host defense mechanisms are encouraged. Lentinan can also improve immune cell reactivity and activate cytokines, hormones, and/or other biologically active substances to secrete. Lentinan increases the resistance of the body to malignant transformation by these properties [11]. Lentinan therapy has also been shown to inhibit prostaglandin synthesis, which often leads to a slowing of the differentiation of T lymphocytes and inhibition of Treg cell activities, in patients suffering from stomach cancer [38]. Increased levels of activated and cytotoxic T lymphocytes in spleen and peripheral cell mononuclear blood stimulation were also observed in generating interleukin 1α (IL-1α), IL-1β, and TNF-α [39]. Certain tumor forms have demonstrated the ability of lentinan in stimulating IL-1 release [40]. In addition to the indirect action, most polysaccharides had direct effects on cancer cells. Many researches about the tumor cell proliferation and/or apoptotic deaths in vitro and in vivo indicate that polysaccharides inhibit tumor cell growth [41]. The modulation of NF-β activity is one of the best-described mechanisms for direct anticancer action of polysaccharides derived from *Basidiomycetes*. Most types of cancer have excessive activation of NF-β. Effective NF-α encourages the development of tumors by stimulating gene transcription, inhibiting cell proliferation, or promoting angiogenesis and metastasis [42]. Polysaccharides have been proven to inhibit NF-α inhibitory phosphorylation and/or degradation [43], which prevents the transcription factor from being activated and therefore its subordinate gene expression [44]. Polysaccharides can influence cancer cells in other ways, in addition to NF-β pathway modulation. The polysaccharide protein complex derived from *Trametes versicolor* as the PSP is an

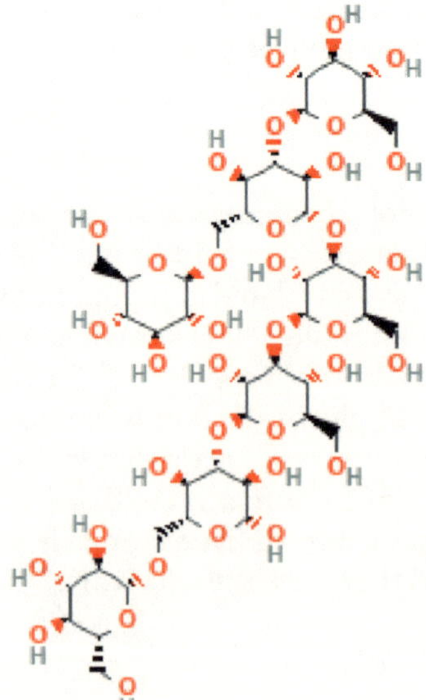

Figure 4.
Chemical structure (2D).

excellent example of this. It was shown that in the leukemia cells U-937 and in the breast cancer cells MDA-MB-231, PSP induced the arrest of cells at G1/S and G2/M restrictive points and inhibited antiapoptotic proteins that caused cell division repression and increased apoptosis [45]. In leukemia cells HL-60, however, the effect of PSP was similar by a decrease of NF-β and ERK kinase expression [46]. In oriental medicine, it is a fundamental principle to control the whole body's homeostasis and return the patient to its normal state [47].

6. Conclusions

Polysaccharides' anticancer properties depend on sugar composition [48], molecular weight [49], water solubility [1], glucose relation [25], tertiary structure [48], branching frequency and shape [41], chemical modification [40], and ligand presence [38]. Scientific approaches to mushroom compounds have allowed the isolation of many of the important active substances used in lifestyle disease prevention and treatment, including cancer. The immune system was strengthened by various polysaccharides from different mushroom varieties. Their ability to stimulate the host's immune system, rather than direct cytotoxicity, all has demonstrated strong antitumor activity. Chemotherapy or radiation therapy seem to withstand and compatible mushroom polysaccharides. Nonetheless, there are urgent needs to be studied that describe the molecular mechanism of mushroom polysaccharides such as receptors and downstream events induced by these polymers being bound to their target cells.

Author details

Moyen Uddin Pk[1,2,3,4,5]*, Rumana Pervin[2], Jabin Jahan[2], Rabiul Islam Talukder[3], Sourav Ahmed[3] and Matiar Rahman[2]

1 Institute of Biological Science, Rajshahi University, Bangladesh

2 Biochemistry and Molecular Biology, Rajshahi University, Bangladesh

3 Biochemistry, Primeasia University, Bangladesh

4 Biochemistry, Independent University, Bangladesh

5 Clinical Biochemistry, Anwer Khan Modern Medical College and Hospital Ltd., Bangladesh

*Address all correspondence to: biomoyen@gmail.com

References

[1] Ferreira ICFR, Vaz JA, Vasconcelos MH, Martins A. Compounds from wild mushrooms with antitumor potential. Anti-Cancer Agents in Medicinal Chemistry. 2010;**10**(5):424-436. DOI: 10.2174/187152061109050424

[2] Byerrum RU, Clarke DA, Lucas EH, Ringler RL, Stevens JA, Stock CC. Tumor inhibitors in *Boletus edulis* and other holobasidiomycetes. Antibiotics and chemotherapy (Northfield). 1957;**7**(1):1-4

[3] Papaspyridi L-M, Aligiannis N, Topakas E, Christakopoulos P, Skaltsounis A-L, Fokialakis N. Submerged fermentation of the edible mushroom *Pleurotus ostreatus* in a batch stirred tank bioreactor as a promising alternative for the effective production of bioactive metabolites. Molecules. 2012;**17**(3):2714-2724. DOI: 10.3390/molecules17032714

[4] Wachtel-Galor S, Yuen J, Buswell JA, Benzie IFF. *Ganoderma lucidum* (Lingzhi or Reishi): A medicinal mushroom. In: Benzie IFF, Wachtel-Galor S, editors. Herbal Medicine: Biomolecular and Clinical Aspects. 2nd ed. Boca Raton (FL): CRC Press/Taylor & Francis; 2011

[5] Chan GC-F, Chan WK, Sze DM-Y. The effects of β-glucan on human immune and cancer cells. Journal of Hematology & Oncology. 2009;**2**:25. DOI: 10.1186/1756-8722-2-25

[6] Kasapis S, Morris ER, Gross M, Rudolph K. Solution properties of levan polysaccharide from *Pseudomonas syringae* pv. phaseolicola, and its possible primary role as a blocker of recognition during pathogenesis. Carbohydrate Polymers. 1994;**23**(1):55-64. DOI: 10.1016/0144-8617(94)90090-6

[7] Lindequist U, Niedermeyer THJ, Jülich W-D. The pharmacological potential of mushrooms. Evidence-based Complementary and Alternative Medicine. 2005;**2**(3):285-299. DOI: 10.1093/ecam/neh107

[8] Cui SW. Food Carbohydrates. Boca Raton: CRC Press; 2005. DOI: 10.1201/9780203485286

[9] Miyazaki T, Nishijima M. Studies on fungal polysaccharides. XXVII. Structural examination of a water-soluble, antitumor polysaccharide of *Ganoderma lucidum*. Chemical & Pharmaceutical Bulletin. 1981;**29**(12):3611-3616. DOI: 10.1248/cpb.29.3611

[10] Rincão VP. Polysaccharide and extracts from *Lentinula edodes*: Structural features and antiviral activity. Virology Journal. 2012;**9**:37. DOI: 10.1186/1743-422X-9-37

[11] Staniszewska J, Szymański M, Ignatowicz E. Antitumor and immunomodulatory activity of *Inonotus obliquus*. Herba Polonica. 2017;**63**(2):48-58. DOI: 10.1515/hepo-2017-0013

[12] Varki A, Cummings R, Esko J, editors. Principles of structural analysis and sequencing of glycans. Essentials of Glycobiology. Cold Spring Harbor (NY): Cold Spring Harbor Laboratory Press; 1999. Chapter 38. Available from: https://www.ncbi.nlm.nih.gov/books/NBK20706/

[13] Mizuno T. The extraction and development of antitumor-active polysaccharides from medicinal mushrooms in Japan (review). International Journal of Medicinal Mushrooms. 1999;**1**(1):9-29

[14] Tomoda M, Gonda R, Kasahara Y, Hikino H. Glycan structures of ganoderans b and c, hypoglycemic glycans of *Ganoderma lucidum* fruit bodies. Phytochemistry.

1986;**25**(12):2817-2820. DOI: 10.1016/S0031-9422(00)83748-6

[15] Huang S, Li J, Li Y, Wang Z. Purification and structural characterization of a new water-soluble neutral polysaccharide GLP-F1-1 from *Ganoderma lucidum*. International Journal of Biological Macromolecules. 2011;**48**(1):165-169. DOI: 10.1016/j.ijbiomac.2010.10.015

[16] Pk MMU, Islam MS, Pervin R, Dutta S, Talukder RI, Rahman M. Optimization of extraction of antioxidant polysaccharide from *Pleurotus ostreatus* (Jacq.) P. Kumm and its cytotoxic activity against murine lymphoid cancer cell line. PLOS One. 2019;**14**(1):e0209371. DOI: 10.1371/journal.pone.0209371

[17] Wu J-Y. Anti-cancer effects of protein extracts from *Calvatia lilacina*, *Pleurotus ostreatus* and *Volvariella volvacea*. Evidence-based Complementary and Alternative Medicine. 2011;**2011**:982368. DOI: 10.1093/ecam/neq057

[18] Cao X-Y, Liu J-L, Yang W, Hou X, Li Q-J. Antitumor activity of polysaccharide extracted from *Pleurotus ostreatus* mycelia against gastric cancer in vitro and in vivo. Molecular Medicine Reports. 2015;**12**(2):2383-2389. DOI: 10.3892/mmr.2015.3648

[19] González-Palma I. Evaluation of the antioxidant activity of aqueous and methanol extracts of *Pleurotus ostreatus* in different growth stages. Frontiers in Microbiology. 2016;7:1099. DOI: 10.3389/fmicb.2016.01099

[20] Jayakumar T, Ramesh E, Geraldine P. Antioxidant activity of the oyster mushroom, *Pleurotus ostreatus*, on CCl(4)-induced liver injury in rats. Food and Chemical Toxicology. 2006;**44**(12):1989-1996. DOI: 10.1016/j.fct.2006.06.025

[21] Vamanu E. Biological activities of the polysaccharides produced in submerged culture of two edible *Pleurotus ostreatus* mushrooms. Journal of Biomedicine and Biotechnology. 2012;**2012**:565974. DOI: 10.1155/2012/565974

[22] Han S-R, Kim K, Lim K-O, Biological activity T-JO. Analysis of different solvent extracts from *Pleurotus ostreatus*. Indian Journal of Science and Technology. 2015;**8**(26):1-8. DOI: 10.17485/ijst/2015/v8i26/80610

[23] Baby S, Johnson AJ, Govindan B. Secondary metabolites from *Ganoderma*. Phytochemistry. 2015;**114**:66-101. DOI: 10.1016/j.phytochem.2015.03.010

[24] Chen H-S. Studies on the immunomodulating and anti-tumor activities of *Ganoderma lucidum* (Reishi) polysaccharides. Bioorganic & Medicinal Chemistry. 2004;**12**(21):5595-5601. DOI: 10.1016/j.bmc.2004.08.003

[25] Gao Y. Antitumor activity and underlying mechanisms of ganopoly, the refined polysaccharides extracted from *Ganoderma lucidum*, in mice. Immunological Investigations. 2005;**34**(2):171-198

[26] Suarez-Arroyo IJ. Anti-tumor effects of *Ganoderma lucidum* (reishi) in inflammatory breast cancer in in vivo and in vitro models. PLOS One. 2013;**8**(2):e57431. DOI: 10.1371/journal.pone.0057431

[27] Aguirre D. Bcl-2 and CCND1/CDK4 expression levels predict the cellular effects of mTOR inhibitors in human ovarian carcinoma. Apoptosis. 2004;**9**:797-805. DOI: 10.1023/B:APPT.0000045781.46314.e2

[28] Willems L, Tamburini J, Chapuis N, Lacombe C, Mayeux P, Bouscary D. PI3K and mTOR signaling pathways in cancer: New data on targeted therapies. Current Oncology Reports. 2012;**14**(2):129-138. DOI: 10.1007/s11912-012-0227-y

[29] Liang Z. *Ganoderma lucidum* polysaccharides prevent palmitic acid-evoked apoptosis and autophagy in intestinal porcine epithelial cell line via restoration of mitochondrial function and regulation of MAPK and AMPK/Akt/mTOR signaling pathway. International Journal of Molecular Sciences. 2019;**20**(3):478. DOI: 10.3390/ijms20030478

[30] Lobo V, Patil A, Phatak A, Chandra N. Free radicals, antioxidants and functional foods: Impact on human health. Pharmacognosy Reviews. 2010;**4**(8):118-126

[31] Tan BL, Norhaizan ME, Liew WP, Sulaiman Rahman H. Antioxidant and oxidative stress: A mutual interplay in age-related diseases. Frontiers in Pharmacology. 2018;**9**:1162. DOI: 10.3389/fphar.2018.01162

[32] Hsieh T-C, Wu JM. Suppression of proliferation and oxidative stress by extracts of *Ganoderma lucidum* in the ovarian cancer cell line OVCAR-3. International Journal of Molecular Medicine. 2011;**28**(6):1065-1069. DOI: 10.3892/ijmm.2011.788

[33] Dai S, Liu J, Sun X, Wang N. *Ganoderma lucidum* inhibits proliferation of human ovarian cancer cells by suppressing VEGF expression and up-regulating the expression of connexin 43. BMC Complementary and Alternative Medicine. 2014;**14**:434. DOI: 10.1186/1472-6882-14-434

[34] Lemieszek M, Rzeski W. Anticancer properties of polysaccharides isolated from fungi of the Basidiomycetes class. Contemporary Oncology (Pozn). 2012;**16**(4):285-289. DOI: 10.5114/wo.2012.30055

[35] Chihara G, Maeda Y, Hamuro J, Sasaki T, Fukuoka F. Inhibition of mouse sarcoma 180 by polysaccharides from *Lentinus edodes* (Berk.) sing. Nature. 1969;**222**(5194):687-688. DOI: 10.1038/222687a0

[36] Zhang P, Cheung PCK. Evaluation of sulfated *Lentinus edodes* alpha-(1-->3)-D-glucan as a potential antitumor agent. Bioscience, Biotechnology, and Biochemistry. 2002;**66**(5):1052-1056. DOI: 10.1271/bbb.66.1052

[37] Bacil ED, Mazzardo Júnior O, Rech CR, Legnani RF, de Campos W. Physical activity and biological maturation: A systematic review. Revista Paulista de Pediatria. 2015;**33**(1):114-121. DOI: 10.1016/j.rpped.2014.11.003

[38] Mizuno M, Nishitani Y. Immunomodulating compounds in Basidiomycetes. Journal of Clinical Biochemistry and Nutrition. 2013;**52**(3):202-207. DOI: 10.3164/jcbn.13-3

[39] Suga T, Maeda YY, Uchida H, Rokutanda M, Chihara G. Macrophage-mediated acute-phase transport protein production induced by lentinan. International Journal of Immunopharmacology. 1986;**8**(7):691-699. DOI: 10.1016/0192-0561(86)90004-4

[40] Bao X, Duan J, Fang X, Fang J. Chemical modifications of the (1-->3)-alpha-D-glucan from spores of *Ganoderma lucidum* and investigation of their physicochemical properties and immunological activity. Carbohydrate Research. 2001;**336**(2):127-140. DOI: 10.1016/s0008-6215(01)00238-5

[41] Zhang M, Cui SW, Cheung PCK, Wang Q. Antitumor polysaccharides from mushrooms: A review on their isolation process, structural characteristics and antitumor activity. Trends in Food Science & Technology. 2007;**18**(1):4-19. DOI: 10.1016/j.tifs.2006.07.013

[42] Ohno N, Miura NN, Nakajima M, Yadomae T. Antitumor 1,3-beta-glucan from cultured fruit body of *Sparassis crispa*. Biological & Pharmaceutical Bulletin. 2000;**23**(7):866-872. DOI: 10.1248/bpb.23.866

[43] Kimura T. Natural products and biological activity of the pharmacologically active cauliflower mushroom *Sparassis crispa*. BioMed Research International. 2013;**2013**:982317. DOI: 10.1155/2013/982317

[44] Yoshioka Y, Ikekawa T, Noda M, Fukuoka F. Studies on antitumor activity of some fractions from basidiomyces. I. An antitumor acidic polysaccharide fraction of *P. ostreatus* (Fr.) Quél. Chemical & Pharmaceutical Bulletin. 1972;**20**(6):1175-1180. DOI: 10.1248/cpb.20.1175

[45] Chow LWC, Lo CSY, Loo WTY, Hu X, Sham JST. Polysaccharide peptide mediates apoptosis by up-regulating p21 gene and down-regulating cyclin D1 gene. The American Journal of Chinese Medicine. 2003;**31**(1):1-9. DOI: 10.1142/S0192415X03000758

[46] Hsieh TC, Wu P, Park S, Wu JM. Induction of cell cycle changes and modulation of apoptogenic/anti-apoptotic and extracellular signaling regulatory protein expression by water extracts of I'm-Yunity (PSP). BMC Complementary and Alternative Medicine. 2006;**6**:30. DOI: 10.1186/1472-6882-6-30 [Published: 11 September 2006]

[47] Chihara G. Recent progress in immunopharmacology and therapeutic effects of polysaccharides. Developments in Biological Standardization. 1992;**77**:191-197

[48] Mizuno T, Saito H, Nishitoba T, KaWagishi H. Antitumor-active substances from mushrooms. Food Reviews International. 1995;**11**(1):23-61. DOI: 10.1080/87559129509541018

[49] Mizuno T. Yamabushitake, Hericium erinaceum: Bioactive substances and medicinal utilization. Food Reviews International. 2019;**11**(1)

Chapter 5

Molecular Mechanism Induced by Beta-Glucans from Maitake to Recover T Cell-Subpopulations during Immunosuppression

Aguilera Braico Diego Maximo and Balogh Gabriela Andrea

Abstract

Breast cancer is the most frequent neoplasia in the world and one of the main causes of death among women. Some of the conventional treatments for cancer are chemotherapy or radiotherapy, knowing that both generate very toxic side effects since they usually affect all cells in active division (healthy or tumoral cells). Therefore, specific treatments are necessary, with therapies aimed at the molecular characteristics of the tumor and its microenvironment. An approach to this could be the search for natural compounds with immunopotentiating capacity and selective toxicity on tumor cells. Recently, immunomodulatory and antitumor activities have been discovered in various fungi. Among them, β-glucans of D-Fraction of *Grifola frondosa* (Maitake) can generate innate and adaptive immune responses, exerting antitumor effects. The reported therapeutic benefits of treatment of breast tumorigenesis with D-Fraction of Maitake require to deepen pharmacological and toxicological studies, in order to guarantee innocuousness and efficacy in the administration to a patient. Therefore, this chapter aimed to elucidate toxicological, pharmacodynamic, and pharmacokinetic aspects of β-glucans from D-Fraction. In this way, we hope to make a significant contribution to the pharmacological knowledge of these bioactive compounds by promoting an immunotherapeutic and antitumor strategy novel agent.

Keywords: beta-glucans, Maitake, D-fraction, toxicological, pharmacodynamic, pharmacokinetic studies, immunosuppression, T-cell lymphocyte

1. Introduction

Grifola frondosa, better known as Maitake, is an edible and medicinal fungus widely known and respected in Eastern countries for thousands of years [1]. It belongs to the *Basidiomycota* division, *Meripilaceae* family, and *Polyporales* order; it grows as a parasite on the bases of deciduous and coniferous trees in forests from Asia, Europe, and eastern North America. It has large annual basidiocarps that can measure up to 1 m in diameter and weigh 20 kg. These are branched and formed by numerous small fan-shaped hats, found themselves imbricated. At the nutritional level, fresh specimens of *Grifola frondosa* have 80% aqueous content, while 22–27% dry weight corresponds to proteins, 50–60% of carbohydrates, and 4% of fats. It has vitamins C, D, and B (B1, B2, B6), niacin, and folic acid. Among its minerals, K, P, and Mg predominate, followed by Zn, Na, Fe, and Ca. As free sugars it has glucose, trehalose, and mannitol. In the formation of basidiocarps, mostly malic acid was identified, but also lactic acid, acetic, formic, citrus, succinic, oxalic, and pyroglutamic acids. The presence of a lectin (N-acetylgalactosamine) capable of agglutinating erythrocytes was also determined. In the early 1980s, Japanese mycologist Hiroaki Nanba identified a fraction present in its mycelium, but also in the fruiting body of *Grifola frondosa* that exhibited greater antitumor activity and significant immunomodulatory effect [2, 3] when administered orally and intravenously, which he called D-Fraction [4, 5]. Since it could be an effective immunomodulator orally, this characteristic made it extremely easy to administer compared, for example, with Shiitake (lentinan) extracts, whose effect was only optimal in intravenous administration [6]. During the 1990s, Nanba and Kubo achieved greater purification of the D-Fraction extract, achieving the MD-Fraction, with superior biological activity [5], highlighting the important antitumor effect of *Grifola frondosa* [7–10]. D-Fraction is insoluble in acid, soluble in alkali, and removable with hot water. Starting with *Grifola frondosa*, a polysaccharide formed by a main chain of branching −1-6-D-Glucoso was placed for every three residues of D-glucose. Glucans are polysaccharides made up exclusively of D-glucose units bound through glycoside bonds, with the glycine being the ones with the greatest therapeutic potential [11, 12]. The purified extract of D-Fraction has main-chain glycogen with branches of −1,3 and the main-chain glucans of the main chain −1,3 with branches −1,6; it also has high molecular weight proteins close to 1,000,000 Da [4, 5].

Numerous fungal compounds—such as D-glucans, proteoglycans, proteins—have been studied in recent years due to their ability to stimulate or inhibit specific components of the immune system [13]. The immunomodulatory effects of D-glucans on the immune system of mammals involves innate and adaptive immune responses, being able to attribute these effects to be a polysaccharide that the body cannot synthesize; the immune system recognizes it as triggering the innate and adaptive immune responses [14] that contribute to the blocking of tumor progression.

Natural killer cells, which are part of innate immunity or first line of defense at birth, are the main weapon of immunosurveillance against tumor development [1], releasing IFN-γ, TNF-α, and GM-CSF in fulfilling its role of smoothing tumor cells. Innate immunity is also composed of monocyte (macrophages) and neutrophils, which, when recognizing foreign agents and put into action various enzymes such as nitric oxide synthase (iNOS), which results in bactericidal intermediaries [13]. Macrophages secrete cytokines (IL-1, IL-6, IL-10, IL-12, TNF-α) capable of modulating innate and adaptive responses, activating, in turn, other macrophages, neutrophils, NK, and T lymphocytes. Tumor activity in NK is enhanced by IL-2, IL-12, and interferons [15]. T cells and NK lymphocytes produce IFN-γ that reinforces the activation of macrophages. The innate response induced by D-Fraction β-glucans involve activation of the protein receptor Dectin-1, which after recognizing these polysaccharides triggers events of phagocytosis and release of cytokines [16, 17]. The extract D-Fraction of Maitake activates the macrophages to secrete IL- 1 [4, 18], IL-12 [8, 17], and TNF-α [19] and stimulates the expression of nitric oxide synthase [20]. In addition to stimulating macrophages, IL-1 promotes the cytotoxicity of splenic T cells, increasing their bactericidal activity [18]. Maitake can stimulate NK cells both in vitro and in vivo, through the increase of IFN-γ and TNF-α in mice [8, 21]. In addition, in macrophages IL-12 secretion associated with NK activation is stimulated by the increased binding to perforins in target cells, increasing tumor lysis [8, 21]. It has been suggested that NK cells are self-activated by the IFN-γ released by themselves [8]. Increased activation of NK was confirmed by increased CD69 expression—NK activation marker—present on the surface of these cells [22]. Subsequent clinical studies in cancer patients revealed that treatment with D-Fraction stimulated and maintained normal activity of NK in peripheral blood [7]. In acquired immunity, which presents as main characteristics specificity and memory [23], D-Fraction of Maitake decreases the expression of the CD69 activation marker of B lymphocytes and stimulates Th lymphocytes, specifically to the Th1 lymphocytes of lymph nodes [8, 19], presenting effects on the balance of Th1 lymphocytes/Th2 lymphocytes [19]. Carcinogenesis has been reported to imply significant imbalance Th1L/Th2L, with a progressive decrease in Th1L (main TLc inducers) and increased Th2L [24]. D-Fraction of Maitake can reverse that imbalance by polarizing the ThL response to Th1L by stimulating the secretion of IL-12 and IL-18 crucial for Th1L activation and blocking Il-1 release important for Th2L activation [19].

2. Immune-restorative capacity of Maitake Pro4X's beta-glucans in immunosuppressed BALB/c females

2.1 Quantification of 1,3-beta-glucans in Maitake Pro4X

The total content of β-1,3 glucans of the purified extract of *Grifola frondosa* (Maitake PRO4X) was quantified through a colorimetric method called Megazyme, a β-glucan commercial kit (Megazyme International Ireland, Bray, Co. Wicklow, Ireland). The samples were performed by triplicate. According to the manufacturer's instructions, 0.1 μl of Exo-1,3-glucanase (20 U/ml) was added to 0.1 ml of sample in sodium acetate buffer at 200 mM concentration and pH 5. The contents were mixed by vortex and incubated at 40°C for 60 min. Subsequently, 3 ml of Buffer GOPOD (glucose oxidase/peroxidase) was added and incubated for 20 min at 40°C. The absorbance value of all samples at 510 nm was read on a Cary 50 Agilent brand UV–Vis spectrophotometer. Finally, the following equation was applied to calculate the concentrations of 1,3-β-glucans:

$$\beta - \text{Glucan } (\%\text{w/w}) = \Delta E \times F/W \times 90$$

where.

ΔE = Absorbance value of the sample at 510 nm.

F = Conversion factor = 100.

W = Sample weight (mg).

Finally, this equation was applied to refer the values with the beta-glucan standard employed in the assay.

$$\frac{\text{Abs Standard (510nm)}}{\text{St. }\beta\text{-glucan}} = \frac{\text{Abs Maitake Pro4X (510nm)}}{\text{Unknown (X)}}$$

St. β-glucan = Standard β-glucan concentration

Unknown (X) = Maitake Pro4x β-glucan concentration

Then, applying the formula, using the values from **Table 1**, the concentration of 1,3-beta-glucans from Maitake Pro4X was obtained.

$$\frac{0.7937}{1.0\ \text{mg/ml}} = \frac{0.7222}{X} \Longrightarrow \boxed{X = 0.91\ \text{mg/ml}\ 1{,}3\ \beta\ \text{glucan in Maitake Pro4X}}$$

2.2 Polarity and solubility of β-glucans from Maitake Pro4X

2.2.1 Polarity of Maitake extract

Evaluation of Maitake Pro4X's polarity by dissolving commercial samples into solvents of increasing polarity. It was checked whether they were soluble, highly soluble, or insoluble. The results are given in **Table 2A**. The results of **Table 2A** on

Sample	Weight (mg)	Absorbance 1 (510nm)	Absorbance 2 (510nm)	Absorbance 3 (510nm)	Average of Absorbance ± S.D	β-glucan (w/v)
Maitake Pro4X	1.00	0.7849	0.7119	0.6698	0.7222 ± 0.058	0.91 mg/ml

Total concentration of 1,3-b-glucans correspond to Maitake Pro4X commercial sample. The test was performed according to the colorimetric method of the Megazyme b-Glucan kit measuring the absorbances of the samples at 510 nm. The Absorbances values indicated in the table are the corrected values referred to the blank of reagents.

Table 1.
Colorimetric quantification of beta-glucan content in Maitake Pro4X.

A

Increase in Solvent Polarity ↓ / Increase in Solubility ↓

Solvents	Maitake Pro4X
N-hexane	Insoluble
Ethyl-acetate	Insoluble
Acetone	Insoluble
Ethanol	Soluble
Methanol	Highly Soluble
Distilled water	Highly Soluble

B

Solvents	Acid/Basic	Maitake Pro4X
Distilled Water	Neutral	Highly Soluble
Hydrochloric Acid	Acid	Highly Soluble
Bicarbonate 7.5%	Basic	Soluble
Oil	---	Insoluble

(A) The solubility of the commercial versions Maitake Pro4X was verified in solvents with increasing polarity. (B) Maitake Pro4X Solubility in acidic or alkaline solvents. The results obtained were recorded as soluble, highly soluble or insoluble.

Table 2.
Polarity/solubility of Maitake.

polarity/solubility of purified Maitake extracts in solvents of increasing polarity showed that both extracts were highly soluble in polar solvents and insoluble in nonpolar solvents. This suggests hydrophilic and polar nature of that compound. Acetone solubility, an aprotic polar solvent (without O—H, N—H links), was differential for both extracts. While Maitake Pro4X proved insoluble, the standard version was soluble. Next, to evaluation the solubility of β-glucans, a 1:4 aqueous dilution of Maitake Pro4X was performed; an aliquot of this dilution was taken in volume similar to the tested for Maitake Standard and dissolved in acetone, being soluble. Dissolution in apolar solvents (n-hexane and ethyl acetate) resulted in the formation of an insoluble upper phase of Maitake (heterogeneous system). In the case of ethanol, both extracts generated a homogeneous system.

2.2.2 Maitake PRO4X solubility

The solubility results of Maitake Pro4X in water-soluble or fat-soluble substances, of an acidic or alkaline nature, are summarized in **Table 2B**. The results of **Table 2A** regarding the solubility of Maitake Pro4X in solvents of acid or alkaline character demonstrated high solubility in acidic pH (hydrochloric acid) and neutral (distilled water) substances. Solubility was observed in bicarbonate 7.5% (m/v) (alkaline pH), with slight ionization of the extract in the form of small whitish precipitates. Maitake Pro4X was insoluble in fat-soluble substances (oil).

2.2.3 pH measurement of Maitake Pro4X

The acidic or alkaline nature of the purified Maitake D-Fraction Pro4X extract from *G. frondosa* mushroom was determined by pH measurement at two different temperatures (20 and 37°C) by the potentiometric method through a pH meter Accumet (Fisher Scientific, USA), using three calibration points and accuracy of pH 0.01. The results of pH indicated an acidic pH for Maitake Pro4X, 5.8 and 5.77, at 20°C and 37°C, respectively. Considering the oral route of administration of beta-glucan compound in mice, we have observed that the pH of Maitake Pro4X is closely related to gastrointestinal organs, the duodenum and colon.

2.3 Role of 1,3-β-glucans from Maitake Pro4X in the mechanism of cell death (apoptosis) mediated by Dectin-1 receptor activation in tumoral MCF-7 cells

2.3.1 Effect of Maitake on human tumor cells with Dectin-1 blocking

The effect of Maitake Pro4X on the feasibility and death of MCF-7 tumor cells was investigated by mediating blocking of Dectina-1 transmembrane receptors with Laminarin. Laminarin, 1,3-β-glucan extracted from *Laminaria digitata*, can specifically bind to the Dectin-1 receptor. It is considered as a Dectin-1 specific blocker. The study indicated that Laminarin connected with ovalbumin OVA could be especially recognized by the Dectin-1 receptor expressed on dendritic cells and macrophage [25]. **Figure 1** illustrates the mechanism of Laminarin blocking the Dectin-1 receptor through activation of certain proteins that inhibit the tumoral cell death induced by Maitake Pro4X alone. This figure's ideas were taken from the publication of Fesel and Zuccaro [26].

In order to study the role of Dectin-1 receptor on cell death induced by Maitake Pro4X, in vitro cultures of MCF-7 cells were treated for 24 h with β-glucans from Maitake Pro4X (367 μg/ml) in the presence and absence of Laminarin (200 μg/ml). The count of living and dead cells was performed in Neubauer's chamber, using

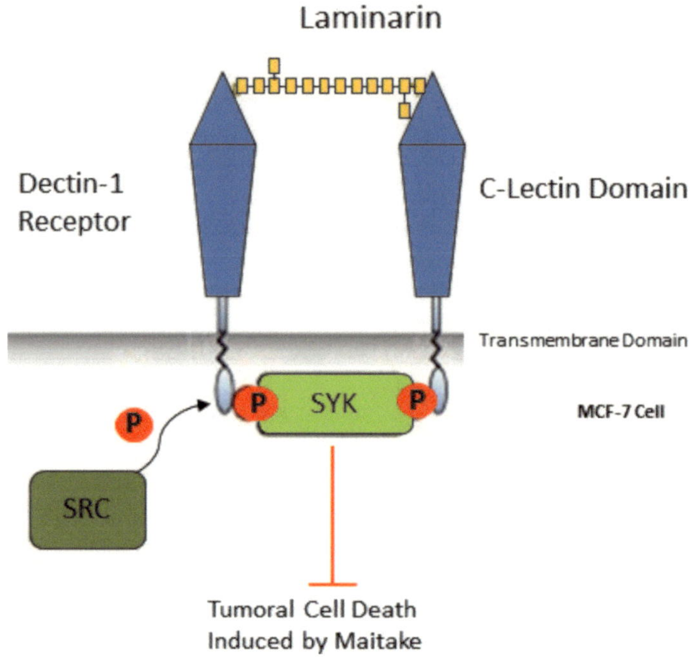

Figure 1.
β-glucan receptor and laminarin. *Upon laminarin binding it is proposed that two Dectin-1 proteins form a receptor co-motif) of both receptor molecules which is subsequently phosphorylated by SRC. Both phosphorylases (SYK, spleen tyrosine kinase) trigger downstream events to block the tumoral cell death induced by Maitake Pro4X. The idea of this graphic was taken from Fesel and Zuccaro [26].*

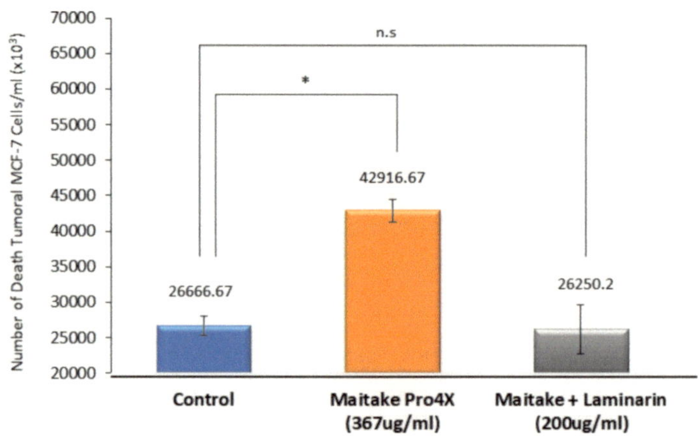

Figure 2.
Effect of tumoral MCF-7 cell death induced by Maitake and dependence of Dectin-1 receptor. *In vitro culture of MCF-7 human tumoral cells was employed to measure the effect of blocking the Dectin-1 receptor (Laminarin 10ug/ml) in the cell death mechanism induced by Maitake Pro4X (5 mg/ml). The experiment was performed by triplicate. The results correspond to mean + 2 standard deviations. In the graphic * means p < 0.05 and n.s means not statistically significant (p > 0.05).*

Trypan blue exclusion technique. The control group was used as untreated. All the experiments were performed by triplicate. The results listed in **Figure 2** about the death of MCF-7 tumor cells demonstrated that treatment with Maitake Pro4X significantly increased (*$p < 0.05$) the death of tumor MCF-7 cells (from 26,666.67 $\times 10^3$ (2.66×10^7) in the control untreated to 42,916.67 $\times 10^3$ (4.3×10^7)). A significant decrease in cell death (*$p < 0.05$) (26,3750 $\times 10^3$ (2.67×10^7)) was found when Dectina-1 receptors were blocked with Laminarin (**Figure 2**).

2.4 Biodistribution of 1,3-beta-glucans from Maitake Pro4X

2.4.1 Biodistribution in oral administration

The uptake of the 1,3-β-glucans from Maitake Pro4X in the various organs was investigated, as well as their accumulation and passage through the blood–brain barrier, after oral intake in BALBc mouse. To achieve this goal, two animals of both sexes were used for each time (n-16), which were administered orally with a single therapeutic dose of 4 μl of Maitake/mouse dissolved in 8 μl of distilled water, corresponding to the therapeutic dose of 5 mg of β-glucans/kg. Subsequently, the mice were treated for 30 min, 1, 2, 4, 7, 16, 24, and 30 h with oral administration with Maitake Pro4X. After that, animals from all groups were induced to death by suffocation with CO_2 in euthanasia chamber and subsequent cervical dislocation. During the autopsy, the hepatic, renal, gastrointestinal (duodenum and colon) organs, lung, and brain removed from each mouse were arranged on a metallic mesh or cell strainer moistened with cold PBS. By means of gentle circular movements with the plunger of the syringe, the organ was disaggregated in the strainer, collecting the homogenization in a falcon tube. In the case of gastrointestinal tissue, its contents were previously removed prior to processing in order to avoid cellular agglomerations. With Pasteur pipette, three washes of 1 ml each of cold PBS were performed to facilitate disintegration; the homogenate remained on ice. With 10 ml syringe and 27 G needle, several passages of aspiration expulsion of tissue filtration were performed, in order to generate complete homogenization and rupture of any cell clusters. Subsequently, it was centrifuged at 1000 rpm for 7 min at 4°C, and the supernatant was discarded. The pellet was resuspended in 4 ml of PBS + SFB 1% and preserved in the freezer at −80°C for subsequent quantification of the glycoprotein extract glucans.

Plasma quantification of 1,3-β-glucans was performed after oral administration of Maitake Pro4X in BALB/c mice. To do time-course curve, two animals were used for each time (condition), making the slaughter of them at 0.5, 1, 2, 4, 7, 10, 16, 24, and 34 h. The determination of 1,3-glucans was performed by the colorimetric test called Glucatell kit (carried out at the Cape Cod Inc. Laboratory, Maryland, USA), which allowed to obtain curves of plasma concentration (pg/ml) vs. post-administration time (h) (**Figure 3**).

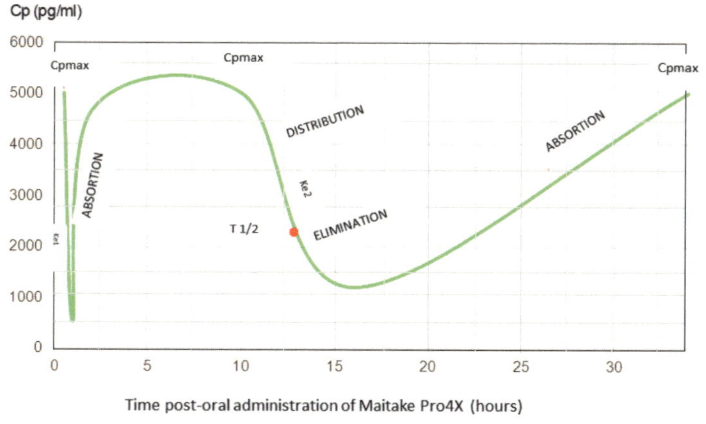

Figure 3.
Plasmatic concentration of 1,3 β -glucans vs time of postoral administration. *The blood was collected during the slaughter of BALB/c mice at pre-established times. Plasma determinations of 1,3-b-glucans were made using the colorimetric method called Glucatell kit. Three peaks of Cpmax were observed following oral administration of Maitake Pro4X (5 mg/kg).*

The pharmacokinetic parameters that were determined are: area under the curve (AUC) Cp vs. time), T 1/2 (half-life time), Cp max (maximum plasma concentration), ke (elimination constant), ka (absorption constant), Ta1/2 (absorption half-life time), Vd (apparent volume of distribution), and Clt (total systemic clearance).

1. **Maximum plasma concentration (Cpmax) and maximum time (Tmax).** The results recorded in **Figure 3** suggest that plasma levels of 1,3-glucans increased rapidly after oral administration, presenting three peaks of maximum plasma concentration:

    a. First peak Cpmax >5000 pg./ml at half an hour after oral administration of Maitake

    b. Second peak Cpmax >5000 pg./ml between 2 and 10 h of oral administration of Maitake

    c. Third peak Cpmax >5000 pg./ml at 34 h of oral administration of Maitake

After the first peak Cpmax, plasma levels of 1,3-glucans fell sharply, resulting in a new Cpmax peak between 2 and 10 h. From 10 h., there was a gradual decrease in the concentration of 1.3-β-glucans. However, after 16 h, a progressive growth of the concentration of 1,3-β-glucans began again, reaching a third peak Cpmax at 34 h after oral administration.

2. **Elimination speed constant (Ke).** The results recorded in **Figure 3** suggest that the removal of 1,3-β-glucans correspond to a first-order kinetic (mono-compartmental) model. The first Ke1 constant has a 4489/h removal speed and Ke2 has a speed of 0.236/h. This indicates a high elimination speed for the range 0.5 to 1 h and more gradual elimination between 10 and 16 h. The first elimination (Ke1) is 19 times faster than the second (Ke1 × 19 Ke2).

3. **Absorption speed constant (ka).** The ka absorption constant was determined by the residual method, assuming a kinetic model of first order with Ka1 > Ke1. First, to calculate ka1, it was drawn the Elimination line Log Cp vs. 0.86 to 0.94 h. Extrapolation was performed to the axis of the ordered, resulting in a line and −22,011x + 4.8472. The selected absorption Cps corresponded to the times 0.6 h (3850 pg./ml), 0.7 h (2300 pg./ml), and 0.8 h (1350 pg./ml). For each time, the Log Cp value was determined on the semilogarithmic elimination line and −22,011x + 4.8472, resulting in 3.53 (0.6 h), 3.31 (0.7 h), and 3.09 (0.8 h). Applying antilogarithm, the elimination Cp was obtained resulting in 3388.44 pg./ml (0.6 h), 2041.74 pg./ml (0.7 h), and 1230.27 (0.8 h). The absorption constant ka1 was calculated from the slope of the absorption line and −29,301x + 44,359, resulting in ka1 × 6.75/h. It was verified that ka1 > ke1. The second absorption constant ka2 was determined by the residual method, assuming a kinetic model of first order with Ka2 > Ke2. The elimination line Log Cp vs. time was plotted in the interval 13 to 15 h, with its corresponding extrapolation to the axis of ordered, resulting in the line and − 0.1144x + 4.83. The absorption Cp stakes chosen in the oral administration curve correspond to the times 1.2 h (1650 pg./ml), 1.4 h (2850 pg./ml), and 1.6 h (3750 pg./ml).

4. **Absorption half-life time (Ta1/2).** From both ka, the absorption half-life time (ta1/2) was established. Using the expression t1/2–0.693/ka, the ta1 1/2 ×

0.1 h was obtained for ka1, while for ka2, the ta2 1/2 × 1.9 h. These results suggest that the plasma concentration of 1,3-glucans that remains to be absorbed was halved to 0.1 and 1.9 am of oral administration.

5. **Elimination half-life time (T1/2).** From both Ke, the elimination half-life time (t1/2) was set, using the expression t1/2–0.693/Ke. For the range 0.5–1 h, t1 × 2 × 0.15 h, while between 10 h to 16 h, t1 × 2.93 h. The plasma concentration of 1,3-glucans was halved at 0.65 and 12.93 h of oral administration.

6. **Distribution volume (Vd).** The apparent volume of distribution was calculated by the expression "Dose/Cp0." The dose administered to the animals was 120 mg of β-glucans (4 ml Maitake PRO4X). Cp0 was determined by extrapolation with the axis of the ordered (ln Cp) in the range 0.5–1 h. So, for a 20 g mouse, the Vd is 2.55 l/0.02 kg, i.e., Vd is 127 ml/g (127 l/kg), this is a great value for Vd on the mouse.

7. **Clearance total (Clt).** Total systemic clearance (Clt) was determined by the expression Clt -Vd (-Ke). For Ke1, Clt-2,55 l × 4489 h-1-11.45 l/h or 190.78 ml/min), while for Ke2, its Clt is 10.03 ml/min.

8. **Area under the curve.** The area under the curve Cp vs. time reflects the amount of bioavailable compound that reaches the systemic circulation and is capable to produce an effect, as determined by the trapezoidal method, resulting in 0.118 mg.h/ml for the time interval 0–34 h.

The results shown in **Figure 4** about tissue uptake of β-glucans following oral administration suggest that the highest concentrations occurred in the stomach (5.52×10^7 pg.h/ml), duodenum (3.66×10^7 pg.h/ml), and colon (3.44×10^7 pg.h/ml). In addition, we have recorded an important level of uptake in the brain (AUC of 3.77×10^4 pg.h/ml) and lung and to a lesser extent at the liver (1.89×10^4 pg.h/ml) and renal (2.44×10^4 pg.h/ml) level. The area under the tissue biodistribution curve of 1,3-β-glucans for the different organs is indicated in **Figure 5**. The results recorded in **Figure 5A** represents the area under the stomach, duodenum, and colon uptake curve of β-glucans. The highest hepatic uptake (**Figure 5B**) occurs at 7 h (*p < 0.05 vs. 2 h) and the lower at 30 h (with **p < 0.01 vs. 2 h). On the other hand,

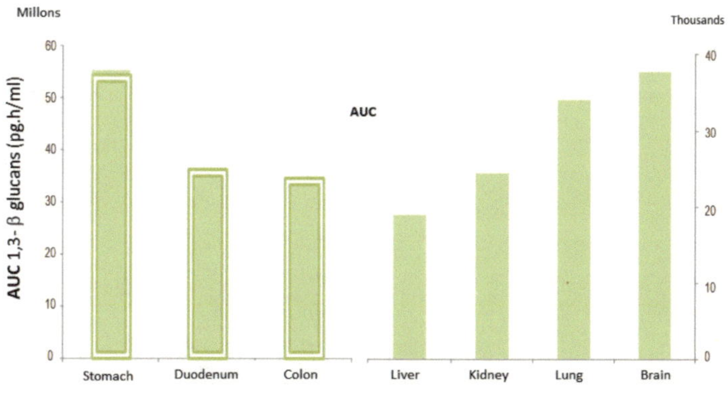

Figure 4.
Mouse tissue biodistribution of 1,3-β-glucans. The catches in the various murine organs were compared between 2 and 30 a.m. after 1,3-b-gucans Maitake Pro4X (5 mg/kg) oral administration. The determinations were made using the colorimetric method of the Glucatell kit. Biodistribution in gastrointestinal organs (stomach, duodenum, colon) was in the order of millions of pg.h/ml, while in others it was thousands of pg.h/ml.

liver uptake at 2 h is significantly higher than that which happens at an equal time in the brain (with $^{*}p < 0.05$). Also, brain uptake at 30 a.m. is significantly less than that occurred at the same lung time (with $^{**}p < 0.01$) (**Figure 5B**).

2.5 Molecular mechanism of dexamethasone in immunosuppression

In order to induce immunosuppression in the experimental murine model, dexamethasone was employed, a synthetic glucocorticoid class of steroid hormones with potent anti-inflammatory and immunosuppressant activities [27]. Dexamethasone-mediated T-cell suppression diminishes naïve T-cell proliferation and differentiation by attenuating the CD28 co-stimulatory pathway [28]. However, the exact molecular mechanism induced by dexamethasone in the immunosuppression is not yet known. **Figure 6** illustrated the possible molecular mechanism of glucocorticoids (GC) such as dexamethasone on immune cells; GCs

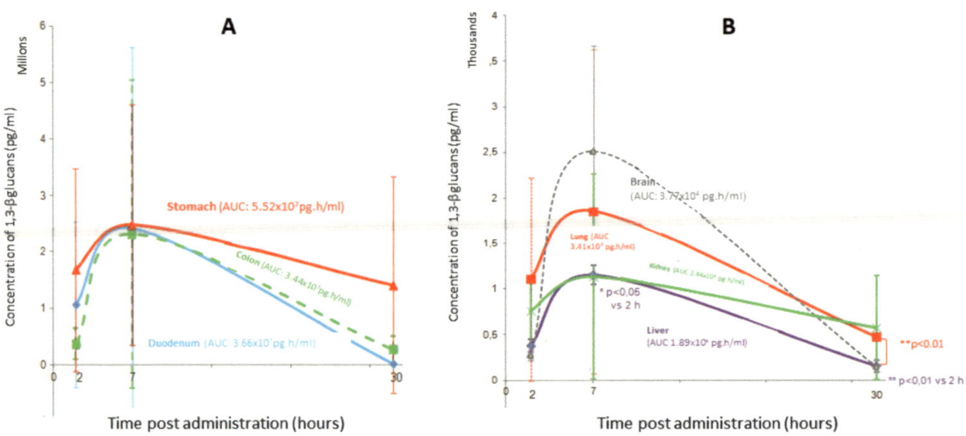

Figure 5
Tissue biodistribution curves of β -glucans. *These correspond to the area under the uptake curve of 1,3-glucans of different murine organs after oral administration of Maitake Pro4X. Mean values +2 standard deviations of: (A) gastric, colonic, and duodenal uptake in millions of pg./ml. (B) Brain, pulmonary, hepatic, and renal uptake in thousands of pg./ml. Significant differences were observed (*p < 0.05; **p < 0.01) between tissue captures and their times.*

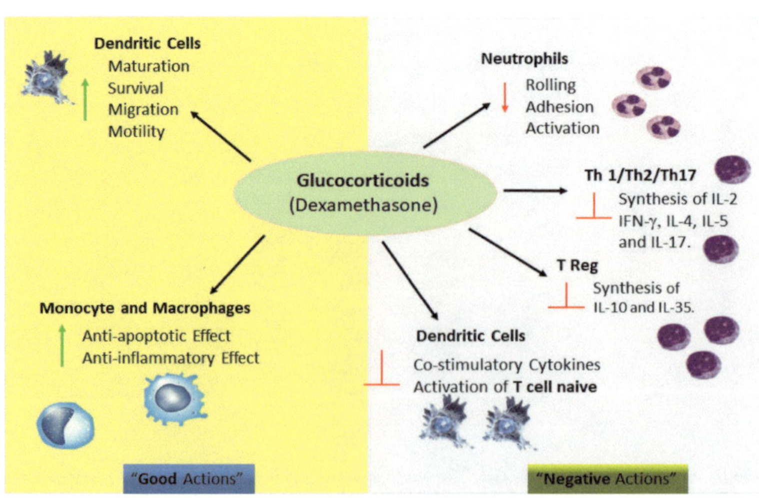

Figure 6.
Glucocorticoid (GC such as dexamethasone) activity on periphery immune cells. GCs act upon almost every immune cell type. This figure was modified from Liberman et al. [29].

promote an anti-inflammatory state on both monocytes and macrophages. GCs prevent monocytes from entering apoptosis and inhibit the liberation of pro-inflammatory mediators by both types of cells. Particularly in macrophages, GCs promote phagocytosis and motility, while they inhibit adhesion, apoptosis, and oxidative burst. They also act upon neutrophil function by inhibiting rolling, adhesion, and activation. GCs act toward dendritic cells by promoting their maturation, survival, migration, and motility, and at the same time GCs inhibit their ability to activate T cells by suppressing the production of pro-inflammatory molecules. A naïve helper T (Th) cell can differentiate into different Th lineages, and GCs exert different actions. They act upon Th1 by decreasing T-bet transcriptional activity and suppressing the production of pro-inflammatory molecules such as IL-2 and IFN-γ. They also suppress GATA3 activity in Th2 cells inhibiting the expression of IL-4 and IL-5. The action of GCs toward Th17 and regulatory T cells is not yet well understood [29] (**Figure 6**).

In order to induce BALBc mouse immunosuppression, 3 g dexamethasone/mouse was administered daily from the beginning to the end of the experimental trial, which lasted approximately for 4 weeks. A suspension of glucocorticoid 0.02% m/v was prepared, for which five tablets of a trademark 0.5 mg were bitten until completely sprayed and suspended in 12.5 ml of 10% aqueous glucose solution. The suspension was prepared weekly and kept in a refrigerator until use. From the suspension of glucocorticoid, daily dainty was administered 15 μl/mouse equivalent to 3 g/mouse/day (0.15 mg de dexamethasone/kg/day).

2.6 Effect of 1,3-β-glucans in the hematology and white blood cell formula

2.6.1 Blood microscopic analysis

Microscopic peripheral blood spread observations were performed for each of the experimental conditions. The blood was collected during the autopsy of the animals and colored with May-Grunwald-Giemsa. Mouse peripheral blood collected during the autopsy of the animals was transferred to Eppendorf tubes containing 0.5% EDTA, at room temperature. A blood smear was performed, placing a drop of blood in the center of a clean slide. A thin film of blood was obtained by means of an object cover (smear). After obtaining the blood smear, it was immediately allowed to air-dry at room temperature, to proceed to its staining. A few drops of methanol were added to fix the preparation, and after evaporation of the preparation, the entire spread was covered with a solution of the May-Grunwald dye for 2–3 min. Subsequently, and unwashed, the Giemsa dye was added for 20 min. Finally, the preparation was washed with distilled water by removing the dyes by trawling and dried at room temperature. **Figure** 7 shows the following conditions:

2.6.2 Healthy control group

Normal red blood cells, clustered platelets, lymphocytes, neutrophils, and monocytes were observed (**Figure** 7 **Superior**). No immature cells were recorded.

2.6.3 Immunosuppressed group

This group presented in his blood abundant large cells, with prominent nucleus, and small and vacuolated cytoplasm (compatible with megakaryocytes); other mice featured megakaryocytes grouped in masse, mastocyte, and PMN basophil and also exhibited monocytes with well-condensed chromatin and megakaryocytes in apparent cell division process. Unevenly sized red blood cells (anisocytosis) were observed (**Figure 7 middle**).

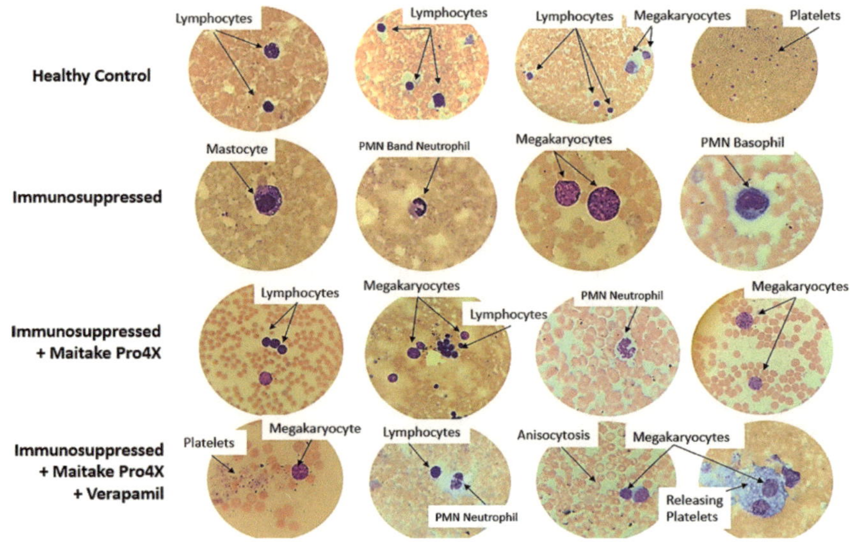

Figure 7.
Blood smear of leukocyte formula. The figure shows the microphotographs from the slides (may-Grunwald-Giemsa x40) indicated in each condition: Healthy control, immunosuppressed in the absence of Maitake Pro4X, immunosuppressed with Maitake Pro4X, and immunosuppressed in the presence of Maitake Pro4X and verapamil.

2.6.4 Immunosuppressed group treated with Maitake

It exhibited mature blood cells such as lymphocytes and polymorphonuclear granulocytes (neutrophils and basophils). In addition, some multinucleated giant cells compatible with megakaryocytes were observed (**Figure 7 middle**).

2.6.5 Immunosuppressed group treated with Maitake + verapamil

Spiculate red blood cells with hypochromia and/or loss of hemoglobin and signs of anisocytosis and hemolysis were observed. In addition, megakaryocytes were released releasing platelets and mastocyte cells in degranulation (**Figure 7 bottom**).

2.7 Flow cytometry studies: expression of CD19, CD3ε, Ly6G, and CD105 molecular markers in immune cells

Flow cytometry studies were performed to analyze the immune-restorative ability of Maitake PRO4X's glucans and recover the immune cell populations with an antigenic expression of CD3ε, CD19, CD105, or Ly6G. Such studies were conducted on murine lymphoid tissues (spleen and lymph nodes) removed during the autopsy of the animals. Maitake's ability to recover immune cell populations in a murine model of immunosuppression was investigated. To do this, 29 healthy BALB/c female mice, 6–8 weeks of age with a weight between 15 and 21 g, were randomly divided into five groups:

1. Condition 1: Healthy control (n = 8)

2. Condition 2: Immunosuppressed (induced by daily administration of *dexamethasone* 0.15 mg/kg) (n = 8)

3. Condition 3: Immunosuppressed with *Maitake PRO4X* (6 mg of β-glucan/kg/Day) (n = 8)

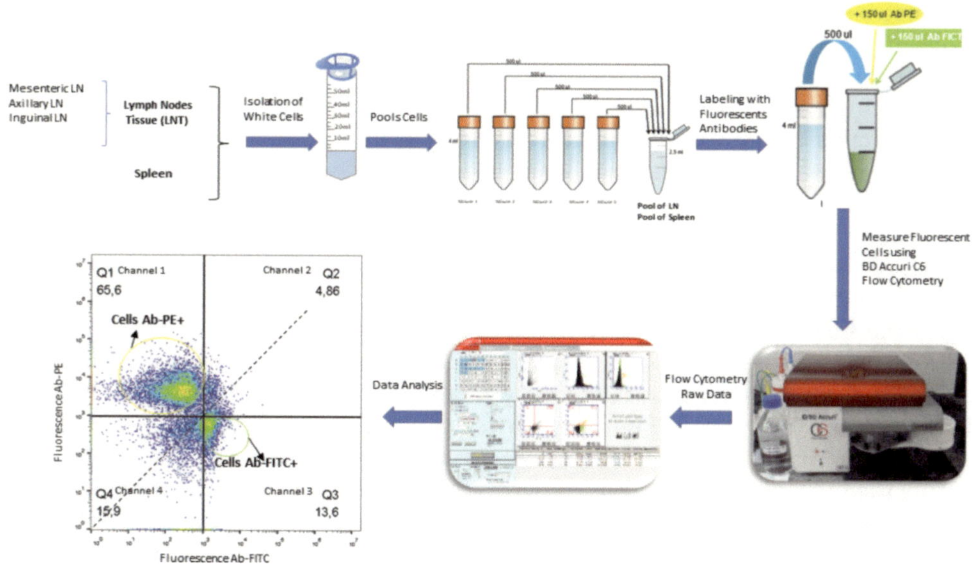

Figure 8.
Lymphoid cell collection. *Mice lymphocytes were obtained from the processing of peripheral lymphoid organs (spleen and murine lymph nodes (mesenteric, axillary, and inguinal LN). The organs were subjected to mechanical disintegration to obtain the cell suspension. After that, a pool of immune cells was performed from each condition studied, cells were stained with specific monoclonal fluorescent anti-mouse antibodies, flow cytometry was performed by triplicate in a BD Accuri C6, and data were analyzed and interpreted as is illustrated in the figure.*

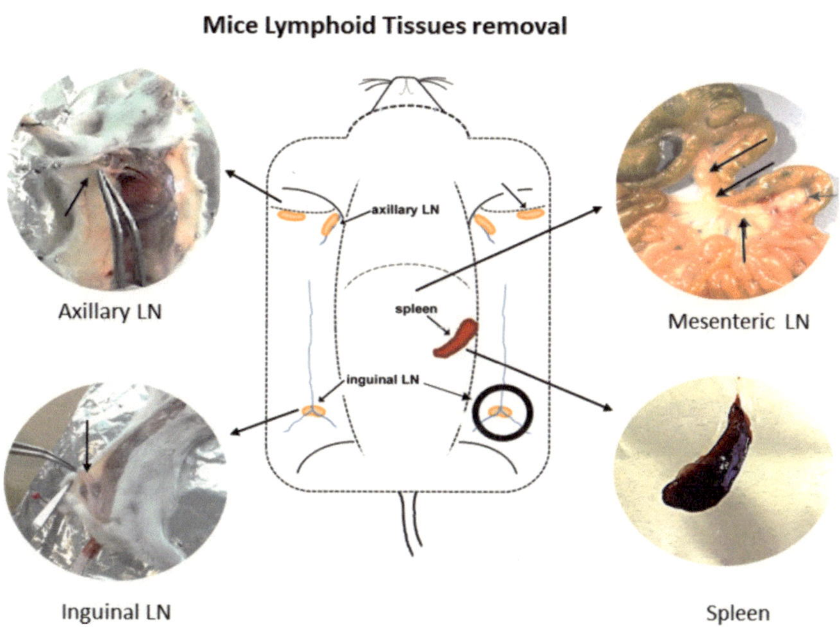

Figure 9.
Removal of peripheral lymphoid organs. *The spleen and lymph nodes (axillary, inguinal, and mesenteric LN) from the BALB/c mice were removed during the autopsy of the animals and subjected to mechanical disintegration to obtain immune cells that were subsequently labeled with the specific antibody to perform flow cytometry.*

4. Condition 4: Immunosuppressed with *Maitake PRO4X* in the presence of a calcium blockage *verapamil* (10 mg/kg/Day) (n = 5)

After 30 days of treatment, all animals were sacrificed using CO_2 asphyxiation camera, and the autopsy was performed in all of them. To perform the flow cytometry studies, immune cells were obtained from peripheral lymphoid organs (spleen and lymph nodes), which were removed during the autopsy of the mice. These organs were placed in a strainer, located in the opening of a falcon tube, to facilitate mechanical disintegration (**Figure 8**). With the plunger of a syringe, gentle circular movements were made resulting in tissue disintegration. The homogenate was collected in the falcon tube. The processing of lymph nodes involved the removal of the inguinal, mesenteric, and axillary nodules (**Figure 9**). Inguinal nodes were observed as small white spots or hardness in the junctions of the blood vessels, while mesenteric nodules were visualized from the unrolling of the small intestine, being observed as a chain of small whitish granules located above the small intestine. From the axillary region, whitish points corresponding to the axillary nodes were removed (**Figure 9**). All three types of nodes were placed in the same strainer after removal, which was previously moistened with cold PBS. The procedure indicated in **Figure 9** allowed to obtain a ganglion homogenate pool, washed three times with 1 ml of cold PBS, and the homogenate was kept on ice during the procedure. With 10 ml syringe and 27 G needle, several suction expulsion passages of filtration were performed to generate complete homogenization and smooth any cell cumulus. Subsequently, the homogenate was centrifuged at 1000 rpm for 7 min using a temperature of 4°C; the supernatant was discarded. The pellet obtained from ganglion cells was resuspended in 4 ml of PBS with bovine fetal serum (FBS 1%), kept in ice until the time of labeled with fluorescent antibodies for flow cytometry. Immune cells were count in Neubauer's chamber before to labeled with fluorescence. In parallel the same procedure was applied with the spleen tissue.

Different populations of immune cells (T lymphocytes, B lymphocytes, natural killer cells, stem cells, PMN granulocytes, and macrophages) derived from the spleen and lymph nodes (**Table 3** and **Figure 10**) were labeled with the following monoclonal anti-mouse fluorescent antibodies:

- Anti-CD3ε-FITC
- Anti-CD19-PE

Monoclonal Antibody Anti-mouse	Clone Number	Label Used	White Cell Type Labelled
CDEε-**FITC** conjugated	145-2011	**CD3ε**	T Lymphocytes (TL) Natural Killer (NK)
CD19-**PE** conjugated	PeCa1	**C19**	B Lymphocytes (BL) Dendritic Cells (DC) Stem Cells (SC)
CD105-**Alexa Fluor** conjugated	MJ7/18	**CD105**	Macrophages Monocytes
Ly6G-**FITC** conjugated	1A8	**Ly6G**	PMN-granulocytes

The different populations of immune cells (T lymphocytes, B lymphocytes, Natural Killer Cells, Stem cells, Polymorphonuclear (PMN) granulocytes and macrophages) from splenic and ganglion tissues were labelled with fluorescent anti-mouse monoclonal antibodies, according to the detail of this table. The conjugated antibody FITC (Fluorescein isothiocyanate), has excitation and emission spectrum peak wavelengths of approximately 495 nm/519 nm, giving it a green color. PE (phycoerythrin)-conjugate fluorescence has an excitation maximum at 564 nm and an emission maximum at 574 nm, giving yellow color. Alexa Fluor (AF) conjugated antibody has the longest wavelength with excitation/emission maximum of 784/814 nm.

Table 3.
Fluorescent anti-mouse antibodies used in flow cytometry.

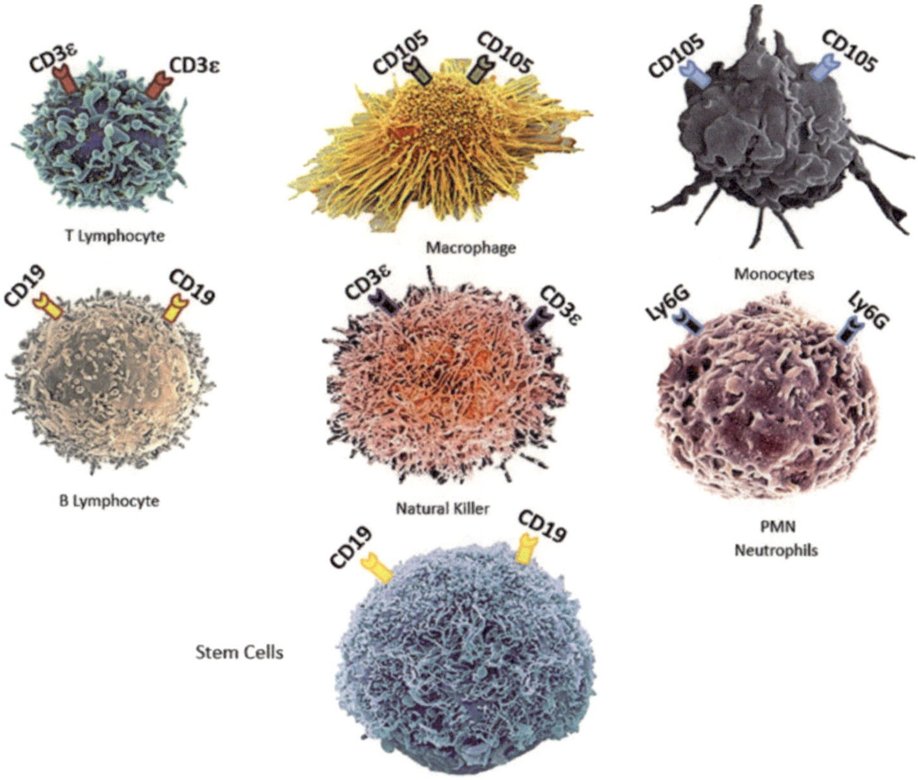

Figure 10.
Molecular markers in flow cytometry. *The immune-restorative effect of Maitake Pro4X in the recovery of immune cells with antigenic expression of CD3ε, CD19, CD105, and Ly6G of the lymph nodes and splenic organs, removed after the sacrifice of the mice, was studied.*

- Anti-CD105-AF
- Anti-Ly6G-FITC

The anti-mouse antibodies used in this study recognize specific markers (surface antigens) of murine immune cells (CD3, CD19, CD105, and Ly6G) and emit fluorescence by being found conjugated with fluorochromes (FITC, PE, and AF), which have different excitation (excitation) and emission wavelengths (Emission) (see **Table 3**). For the fluorescent labeling with the conjugated antibody with PE + FITC, 500 μl of cells from the pellet were taken from the sample pool, and added 150 μl of PE antibody (1:30) plus 150 μl of FITC antibody (1:30) were mixed and incubated in dark for 30 min at room temperature. After that time, the cells were washed twice with 500 μl of cold PBS and centrifuged for 7 min at 1000 rpm. The supernatant was discarded, the cell pellet was resuspended with 400 μl PBS + PFA (paraformaldehyde acid) 1% and kept on ice (always safe from light), until the time of reading on the cytometer, after homogenization of the samples, and according to the manufacturer's instructions. A BD Accuri C6 flow cytometer was used with a blue laser (480 nm) for the excitation wavelength and a red laser (640 nm) for the emission wavelength. The data was acquired on a logarithmic scale and analyzed with the FlowJo software (Tree Star, Ashland, OR, USA) (**Figure 8**).

The flow cytometry results of **Table 4**, **Figures 11** and **12** regarding the recovery of CD3 immune cells suggest that treatment with Maitake Pro4X allows a very significant recovery (**$p < 0.01$) of % T/natural killer lymphocytes (from

6.80 ± 7.08% to 21.09 ± 12.39%) in female BALB/c immunosuppressed with dexamethasone with respect to the immunosuppressed control (**Figures 11A–C** and **12A**). On the other hand, immune-restoration reaches normal values when Maitake treatment is adjuvant with Verapamil (from 21.09 ± 12.39% to 27.04 ± 29.96%) (**Figures 11D** and **12A**). As for the CD19 labeling, the results of

Ganglion Cells	CD3ε (%) (LT/NK)	CD19 (%) (LB/SC)
Healthy Control	51,14 ± 9,85	9,85 ± 2,62
Immunosuppressed (Dexamethasone)	6,80 ± 7,08 (**)	0,0 ± 0,00 (**)
Immunosuppressed with Maitake	21,09 ± 12,39 (**)	1,10 ± 1,67 (**)
Immunosuppressed + Maitake + Verapamil	27,04 ± 29,96 (**)	0,00 ± 0,00 (**)

The percentages obtained by flow cytometry correspond to axillary, mesenteric and inguinal lymph nodes of BALB/c females treated with Maitake Pro4X in the presence of immunological depletion and/or channel calcium blockage. The statistically very significant difference are indicated with (**).

Table 4.
Ganglion CD3ε and CD19 expression.

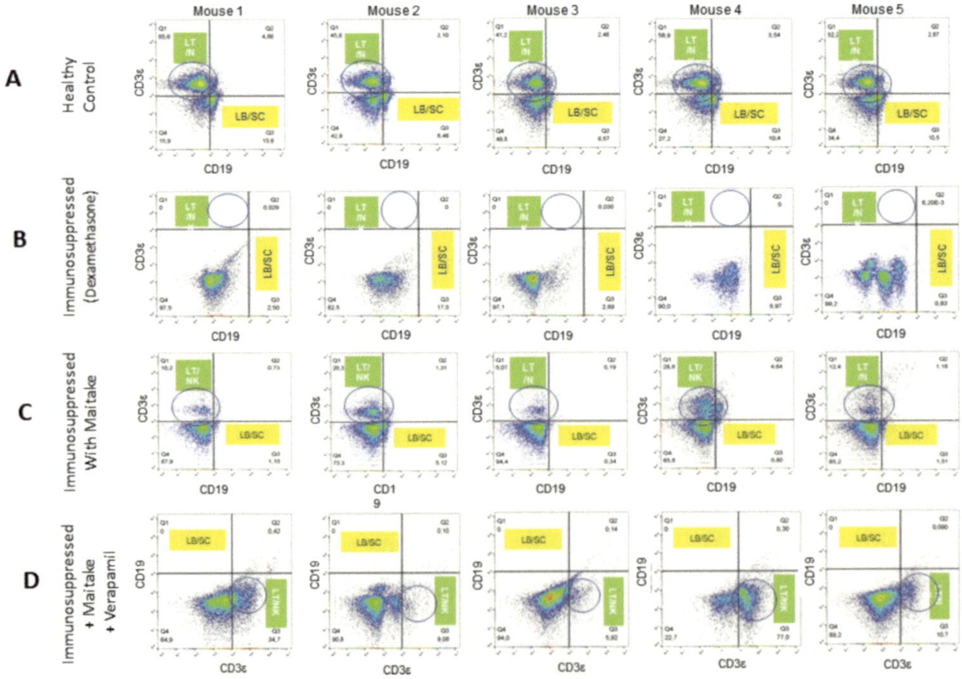

Figure 11.
Expression ganglion CD3/CD19. These correspond to axillary, mesenteric, and inguinal lymph nodes of BALB/c females of four experimental conditions: (A) healthy control group, (B) immunosuppressed condition, (C) immunosuppressed group treated with Maitake, (D) immunosuppressed group treated with Maitake + verapamil.

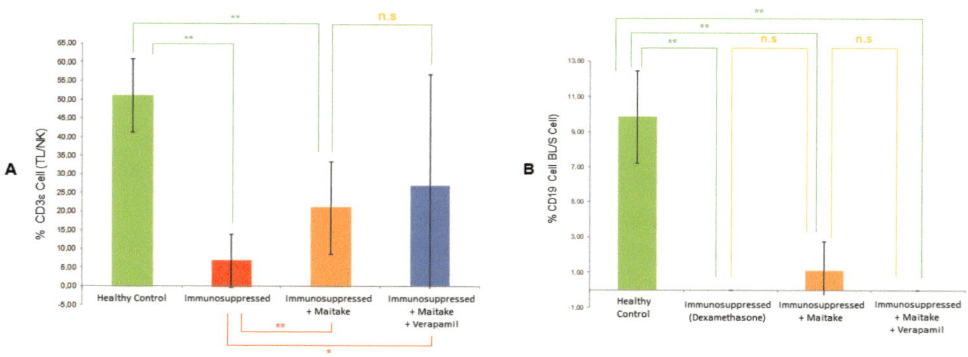

Figure 12.
Maitake's immune-restorative effect on CD3 and CD19 mouse immune ganglion cells. *The cytometric assay was performed on BALB/c females immunosuppressed with dexamethasone. The following are plotted: (A) CD3ε marking with very significant recovery of LT/NK (**p < 0.01) by Maitake effect in the immunosuppressed group and (B) CD19 marking with tendency to recover FROM LBT/SC by Maitake effect (ns, p > 0.05).*

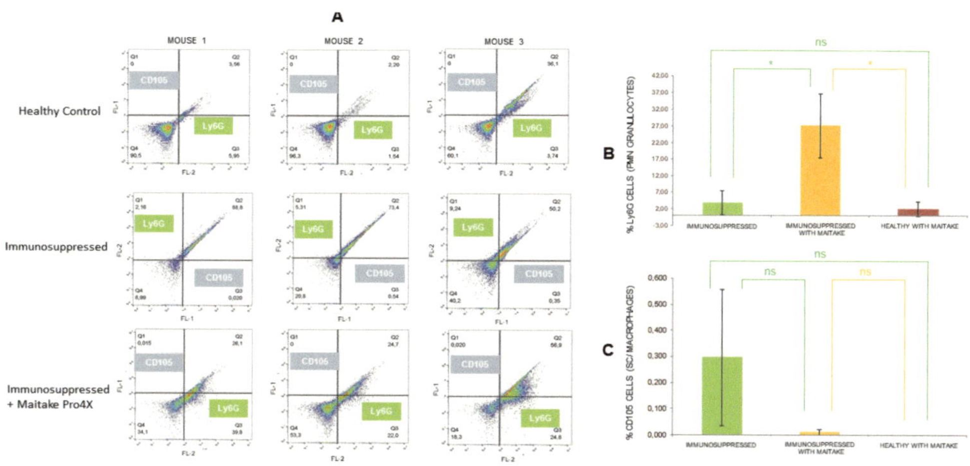

Figure 13.
Ly6G/CD105 mouse ganglion expression. *(A) Flow cytometry charts correspond to axillary, mesenteric, and inguinal lymph nodes of BALB/c females of three experimental conditions: Healthy group, immunosuppressed group alone, and treated with Maitake (B) and (C) Maitake's immune-restorative effect on Ly6G and CD105 immune ganglion cells. The cytometric assay was performed on BALB/c females immunosuppressed with dexamethasone. Graphed: (B) shows Ly6G labeling with significant differences in % of PMN granulocytes (*p < 0.05) and (C) shows the CD105 labeling cells without significant differences in the % of SC (stem cells)/ macrophages cells (ns, p > 0.05).*

Figures 11A–D and **12B** suggest that daily dexamethasone depletes the LB/SC population, while treatment with Maitake Pro4X tends to recover the LB/SC population (from 0.00 to 1.10 ± 1.67) (ns, $p > 0.05$). But this immune-restoration tends to disappear when treatment involves verapamil (from 1.10 ± 1.67 to 0.00 ± 0.00).

The flow cytometry results indicated in **Figure 13A** and **B** regarding the recovery of Ly6G ganglion immune cells suggest that treatment with Maitake Pro4X significantly increases (with $^*p < 0.05$) the % polymorphonuclear granulocytes (PMNG) in the immunosuppressed mice with dexamethasone (immunosuppressed) from 3.88 ± 3.55% to 27.18 ± 9.57%, but does not increase it in healthy mice group. With respect to the CD105 cells, the results shown in **Figure 13A** and **C** suggest that dexamethasone does not induce depletion of % of stem cells (SC)/macrophages, given the not that significant differences (ns, $p > 0.05$) in the level of these cells among the experimental groups.

	CD3ε Splenic Cells (%)	CD19 Splenic Cells (%)
Healthy Control	23.47 ± 7.49	6.90 ± 2.88
Immunosuppressed	16.68 ± 9.17	0.953 ± 0.767
Immunosuppressed + Maitake Pro4X	27.79 ± 3.77	1.34 ± 0.43
	Ly6G Splenic Cells (%)	**CD105 Splenic Cells (%)**
Healthy Control	21.32 ± 15.32	0.06 ± 0.08
Immunosuppressed	18.09 ± 3.01	0.73 ± 0.72
Immunosuppressed + Maitake Pro4X	16.45 ± 4.94	0.12 ± 0.21

The percentages obtained by flow cytometry correspond to murine spleen tissue of BALB/c females treated with Maitake Pro4X in the presence of immunological depletion with Dexamethasone.

Table 5.
Splenic CD3ε, CD19, Ly6G, and CD105 cell expression.

2.7.1 Mouse splenic labeling of CD3 and CD19 cells

Flow cytometry results for splenic immune CD3 and CD19 cells' recovery are listed in **Table 5**. This trial was conducted with three experimental conditions: healthy control, immunosuppressed group alone, and immunosuppressed group treated with Maitake Pro4X. The flow cytometry results suggest that treatment with dexamethasone does not induce a significant depletion of the LT/NK population compared to the other experimental groups (ns, $p > 0.05$). There is a trend of the reduction of LT/NK % per share of dexamethasone and a trend of increased LT/NK by Maitake effect in the immunosuppressed group. Regarding the CD19 labeling (**Table 5**), we observe a significant depletion of the splenic population of LB/SC by dexamethasone (*$p < 0.05$ vs. healthy group) and a tendency to recover that population by Maitake (ns, $p > 0.05$).

As for the immune system, regulating its activation or suppression could contribute to the maintenance of good health. The use of agents that activate host defense mechanisms (immune-stimulators, immuno-suitors, or biological response modifiers) could provide an additional therapeutic tool to conventional chemotherapy [25]. For this reason, many biomedical researches are geared toward the search for new compounds capable of stimulating an immune response in immunodeficient patients, with pathologies such as HIV/AIDS, cancer, or malnutrition [30, 31]. Numerous immunostimulatory substances have been isolated from plants and superior fungi, opening the doors for the development of new drugs [30]. This provides an effective alternative for the treatment of conditions that alter the normal balance of the body's immune response [32, 33].

Within this context, we have investigated the immune-restorative capacity of Maitake Pro4X's glucans in BALB/c females immunosuppressed with dexamethasone. In parallel to immunosuppressive treatment, we treat mice with Maitake glycoprotein extract; it is important to note that no animals perished as a result of immunosuppressive treatment and that clinical signs of toxicity or disease were also not observed.

3. Discussion and conclusions

The antitumor and immunosurveillance properties of D-Fraction of Maitake have been little explored for the application in breast tumor or clinical immunosuppression pathologies. For this reason, this chapter aims to deepen research on the pharmacokinetic and pharmacodynamic aspects of β-glucans from Maitake D-Fraction, as well as their therapeutic effects on immune recovery of specific lymphocyte populations. This is in order to make a significant contribution to the development of new preventive and therapeutic strategies to optimize the pharmacological use of Maitake's glucans.

As part of our experimental studies, we have observed in physicochemical characterization assays that the pH value of purified Maitake extracts measured at 20°C (ambient temperature) and 37°C (body temperature) resulted to be acidic with pH 5.8 for Maitake Pro4X. Moreover, this product was soluble in polar solvents (water, methanol, ethanol) and insoluble in apolar solvents (n-hexane, ethyl acetate), demonstrating its hydrophilic and polar nature. We also observe an inverse relationship between the proteoglycan concentration and its solubility in polar solvents (such as acetone), resulting in insoluble in acetone. The above suggests that D-Fraction of Maitake has hydrophilic and polar nature. The pH similarity of the product to the gastrointestinal pH suggests a good absorption at that level, which is associated with the biodistribution results shown here for oral administration.

The high molecular weight of β-glucans from Maitake extract suggests the great difficulty of these molecules in crossing biological membranes by simple diffusion, requiring a specific receptor after entering the systemic circulation, in order to trigger their molecular action mediated by second intracellular messengers. Nakashima et al. [34] in agreement with Brown et al. [35, 36] had reported that the Dectina-1 membrane receptor recognizes "glucans" with links "β-1,3" and/or "β-1.6" present on the fungal walls, proposing that receptor as a new receptor and as a therapeutic target for the immunomodulatory effects of glucan compounds.

Another of our in vitro assays showed that the treatment of MCF-7 breast tumor cells with Maitake + laminarin (Dectin-1 inhibitor) significantly reduced the effect of cell death triggered by Maitake ($p < 0.05$). These results suggest a greater affinity of Dectina-1 receptors with laminarin than Maitake's glucans. In addition, a likely laminarin-Dectin-1 complex would prevent the binding of β-glucans to the tumor receptor by blocking the mechanism that leads to programmed cell death.

As for our pharmacokinetic parameter studies in oral administration, we have observed three peaks of plasma concentration of 1.3-β-glucans with a maximum peak that was recorded half an hour after administration (followed by an abrupt decline). The second peak was recorded between 2 and 10 h thereafter and the last at 34 h after oral administration of Maitake Pro4X-glucans (5 mg/Kg). The results of our trials suggest that the plasma removal (clearance) of 1.3-β-glucans corresponds to a first-order kinetic model (mono-compartmental), obtaining a very rapid first plasma disappearance initiated at half an hour and a second more gradual elimination at 10 h later. Hong et al. [37] have reported that orally administered β-1,3-glucans are transported by macrophages to the spleen, lymph nodes, and bone marrow, implying a possible plasma reduction of the compound. For our part, we have observed that the absorption of the compound was higher than the elimination of the compound and that the volume of the distribution obtained was very high (127 ml/g). These results would indicate the extensive distribution of glucans in tissues and poor plasma protein binding. So that probably the 1,3-β-glucans could be found mostly in their "free" form in blood circulation, being able to diffuse the extravascular compartments, to interact with their receptors, and to trigger a biological response.

Moreover, in the hematological analysis of mouse peripheral blood in various experimental conditions, we have observed that the dexamethasone (immunodepleted) group had many giant cells of immature appearance compatible with megakaryocytes, while the condition with Maitake + dexamethasone group presented low number of immature cells, in addition to increasing number of lymphocytes, PMN neutrophils, basophils, and some megakaryocytes. In turn, the group dexamethasone + verapamil + Maitake exhibited megakaryocytes and mast cells in degranulation [38]. The healthy control group did not have immature cells, with clustered platelets, lymphocytes, neutrophils, and monocytes observed. Our microscopic observations suggest that as a result of immunodepletion in mice by dexamethasone, large immature cells are recruited into the bloodstream, while concomitant treatment with Maitake could contribute to cell maturation, corroborated by the presence of mature basophil cells, lymphocytes, and polymorphonuclear granulocytes. These results suggest that Maitake's glucans could induce cellular maturation leading to immune-restoration. However, when treatment with Maitake involves calcium receptor blockage, its immunosurveillance capacity would be reduced, highlighting the dependence of extracellular calcium. Estrada et al. [39] have reported that the "glucans" increase the proliferative capacity of cultured lymphocytes treated with dexamethasone, reversing the immunosuppressive effect of glucocorticoid, suggesting the ability of the glucans to restore significantly specific and non-specific immune parameters in both cell cultures and animals treated with dexamethasone. For their part, Kotthoff et al. [40] have reported that antigen-presenting cells generated in the presence of dexamethasone have reduced the ability to stimulate the proliferation of T cells, while treatment with β-glucans induces the expression CD69 T-cell maturation markers and promotes Syk and STAT3 phosphorylation, with increased IL-10 secretion, while reducing the production of IL-12, IL-23, and TNF-A. Masuda et al. [41] reported, in murine models of tumorigenesis, that MD-Fraction of *Grifola frondosa* could generate systemic immune response, directly inducing the maturation of dendritic cells through a Dectin-1 pathway of the receptor Dectin-1 lectin type C. The therapeutic response of orally administered MD-Fraction was associated with specific T-cell responses of induced systemic tumor antigen through Dectin-1-dependent activation of dendritic cells, (ii) increased T-cell infiltration, and (iii) decreased number of immunosuppressive cells caused by tumors, such as regulatory T cells and myeloid-derived suppressive cells [41]. For our part, the studies of flow cytometry in dyed lymph nodes with CD3ε (LT, NK)/CD19 (LB, SC) suggested that treatment with Maitake allows a very significant recovery ($^{**}p < 0.01$) of the T/natural killer lymphocyte population of immunosuppressed animals with dexamethasone. In turn, concomitant treatment with verapamil would not affect the described immune-restoration but would instead contribute to lymphocyte recovery reaching normal values. So Maitake-induced cellular maturation could be affected by extracellular calcium blockage based on our microscopic results, but recovery of T/natural killer lymphocytes would not be influenced by the ion sequestration. With respect to the LB/SC population, we note that Maitake Pro4X tended to recover that lymphocyte population, but without statistical significance, while joint treatment with verapamil inhibited this trend. The results described support our hypothesis that extracellular calcium sequestration affects some of the functionalities of Maitake's glucans. On another hand, the molecular marker CD105 (for stem cells/macrophages) was found no significant differences in the cell population between the different experimental conditions. Similar results were obtained for ganglion molecular marker CD19 (stem cells/LB) with no significant differences between animal groups. Regarding Ly6G ganglion molecular marker (polymorphonuclear granulocytes), we observe that treatment with Maitake significantly increased the percentage of the cell population in immunosuppressed mice ($^{*}p < 0.05$) but not in healthy animals.

Lin et al. [42] in previous studies reported the ability of Maitake's glucans to activate the biological response in hematopoiesis, promoting bone marrow recovery after injury and stimulating activation of the Maitake forming unit granulocyte and monocyte colonies (GM-CFU), while Kodama et al. [43] have reported that D-Fraction derived from *Grifola frondosa* is able to activate immunocompetent cells such as macrophages and T cells, with modulation of the balance between T-helper lymphocytes 1 and 2. Continuing with our studies at the splenic level, we do not find in the spleen more significant effect of immune-restoration than that described for lymph nodes, prompting the tendency to recover immune populations by Maitake effect. In splenic tissue the CD19 (LB/SC) molecular marker labeling was significantly depleted during treatment with dexamethasone compared to the healthy group treated with Maitake Pro4X (*$p < 0.05$), while treatment with Maitake alone induced only trend in the recovery of B lymphocytes ($p > 0.05$). In another sense, dexamethasone did not induce significant depletion of the splenic CD3 cell population (LT/NK) with respect to the healthy group treated with Maitake, although it tended to reduce LT/NKs, while concomitant treatment with Maitake tended to increase this population. Dexamethasone also did not significantly deplete the splenic Ly6G cell population (PMN granulocytes) and CD105 (SC/macrophages) for the healthy group treated with Maitake. In the splenic CD105 (SC/macrophages), dexamethasone tended to increase that population compared to the healthy group treated with Maitake, while joint treatment with Maitake tended to reduce it. These effects were like those observed for SC/macrophages at the ganglion level. These results suggest greater relevance of the immune-restorative effect of Maitake and immunosuppressant effect of dexamethasone at the ganglion level rather than splenic. Kay and Czop [44] previously reported that dexamethasone stimulates monocyte gluconic receptors and promotes phagocytosis by macrophages of particles of β-glucans. In vivo studies in murine models of immunosuppression showed that dexamethasone (immunosuppressant) promotes the presence of immature immune cells in circulation, while concomitant treatment with Maitake stimulates maturation and cell differentiation (with the presence of polymorphonuclear granulocytes, lymphocytes, and basophilic cells). Extracellular calcium blockage (Maitake + verapamil adjuvant) partially affects the immune-restorative effect for certain lymphocyte populations. Flow cytometry studies demonstrated a significant immune-restorative effect of Maitake at the ganglion level, with recovery from polymorphonuclear granulocytes and LT/NK, while concomitant treatment with verapamil further increased the recovery of LT/NK.

In conclusion, the in vivo studies in murine models of immunosuppression showed that dexamethasone (immunosuppressant) promotes the presence of the high number of immature immune cells in circulation, while the concomitant treatment with Maitake stimulates maturation and cell differentiation (with the presence of polymorphonuclear granulocytes, lymphocytes, and basophilic cells). The extracellular calcium blockage (Maitake + verapamil adjuvant) partially affects the immune-restorative effect for certain lymphocyte populations. Flow cytometry studies demonstrated a significant immune-restorative effect of Maitake at the ganglion level, with recovery from polymorphonuclear granulocytes and LT/NK, while concomitant treatment with verapamil further increased the recovery of LT/NK.

From the in vivo biodistribution studies in murine models, we have concluded that after oral administration, there was increased uptake of the gastrointestinal compound with the predominance of gastric uptake but also important uptake in the duodenum and colon (in the order of millions of pg.h/ml). The presence of β-glucans in the brain allows Maitake's ability to pass through the blood–brain barrier (BHE). The lower relative uptake recorded at the hepatorenal level allows us to conclude a lower rate of inactivation and excretion of the compound, evidenced by the longer circulation time of the compound in the body after a single administration.

In resume, based on the results obtain in this work, we can propose the following putative molecular mechanism on mice (**Figure 14**): After oral administration of 1,3-1,6-β-glucans from Maitake Pro4X, due to its hydrophilic nature and high solubility in the stomach/duodenum with similar Ph, the complex 1,3-1,6-β-glucans are captured

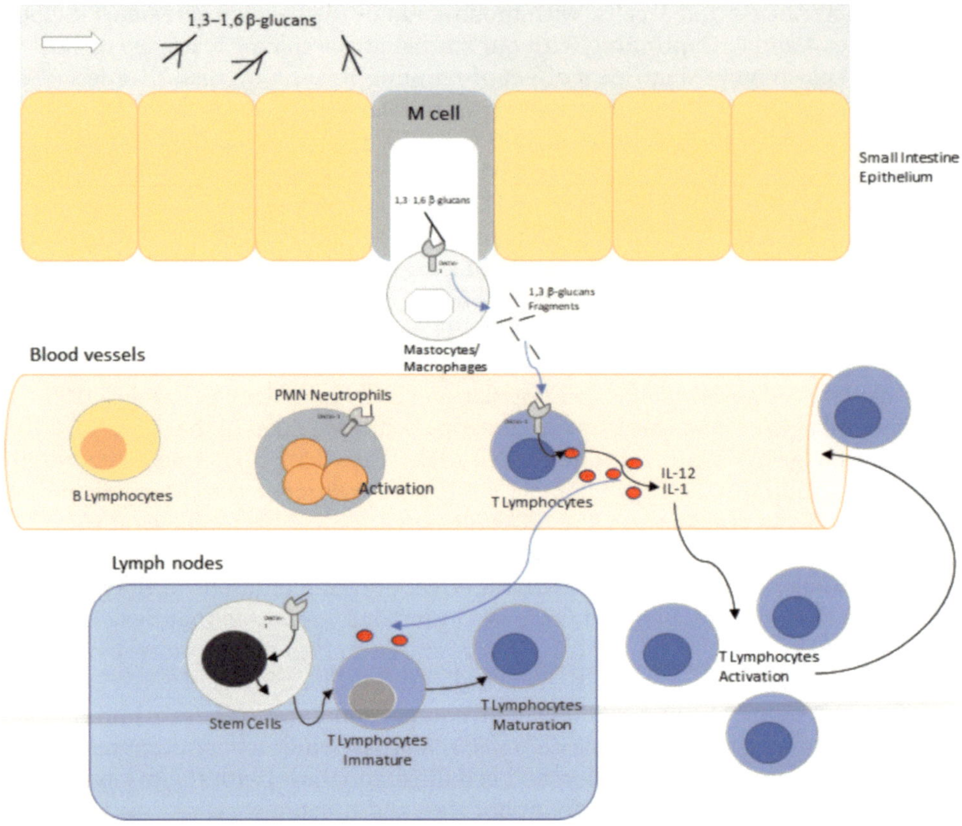

Figure 14.
Putative molecular mechanism induced by 1,3-b-glucans from Maitake Pro4X to revert the immunosuppression situation. *We have demonstrated Maitake's D-fraction's ability to restore specific lymphocyte populations in lymph nodes, including polymorphonuclear granulocytes and LT/NK, as well as induce maturation of T cells on bone marrow and lymph nodes.*

by mastocytes/macrophages through Dectin-1 receptors in M cells in the epithelium from the small intestine; after that, beta-1,3-glucan fragments (are broken in pieces) pass through the blood vessels' endothelium impacting the receptor Dectin-1 on T-lymphocyte cells, stimulating their expression of lymphokines such as IL-12 and IL-1, attracting more T lymphocytes, and helping in the recovery of T-cell population during immunosuppression. On lymph nodes (ganglion cells), β-1,3-glucan fragments stimulated the stem cells to differentiate into TL and mature to reestablish the TL cells on blood circulation due to dexamethasone effect on immunosuppression. The most spectacular action of beta-glucans is the effect on PMN granulocytes especially on neutrophils (the first barrier of defense in the body) (**Figure 14**). In conclusion we can be optimistic to see how promising the beta-1,3-glucan natural compound can be to be applied in immunodepleted situations helping the T cells and PMN granulocytes recover its population through stem cell differentiation, maturation, and activation in order to reestablish a new immune barrier ready to defend the body.

Acknowledgements

We acknowledge the National Council of Research from Argentina CONICET for its support since 2008. We thank Mushroom Wisdom Inc., NY, USA, for their support since 2008 and for providing Maitake Pro4X for all the studies done in this chapter.

We thank Dr. Prof. Eustaquio Souza Días, Laboratório de Cogumelos Comestíveis Biology Department, Universidade Federal de Lavras, Lavras, Brazil, for his help in the quantification of β-glucans in Maitake Pro4X.

We thank Mr. Malcolm Finkelman from the Clinical Development Department at Associates of Cape Cod, Inc., East Falmouth, MA, USA, for his great help in the studies of beta-glucan biodistribution in mouse tissue.

Conflict of interest

The authors declare no conflict of interest.

Thanks

Thanks to the Almighty God, for this chapter and for our lives which is dedicated to Him. Thanks to Dr. Diego Aguilera Braico, my best friend and the most incredible and happy person that I have ever met in Argentina.

Abbreviations

ThL	T-helper lymphocyte
NK	natural killer cells
IFN-γ	interferon gamma
IL-	interleukin
TNF-α	tumor necrosis factor alpha
iNOS	nitric oxide synthase
GM-CSF	granulocyte macrophage colony-stimulating factor
BL	B lymphocytes
TL	T lymphocytes

Author details

Aguilera Braico Diego Maximo and Balogh Gabriela Andrea*
National Council of Research from Argentina CONICET, Bahia Blanca, Argentina

*Address all correspondence to: gbalogh@ichsphila.org

References

[1] Mao GH, Ren Y, Feng WW, et al. Mint: Antitumor and immunomodulatory activity of a water-soluble polysaccharide from Grifola frondosa. Carbohydrate Polymers. 2015; **134**:406-412. DOI: 10.1016/j.carbpol.2015.08.020

[2] Kodama N, Murata Y, Nanba H. Mint: Administration of a polysaccharide from Grifola frondosa stimulates immune function of normal mice. Journal of Medicinal Food. 2004; **7**(2):141-145. DOI: 10.1089/1096620041224012

[3] Kodama N, Asakawa A, Inui A, et al. Mint: Enhancement of cytotoxicity of NK cells by D-fraction, a polysaccharide from Grifola frondosae. Oncology Reports. 2005;**13**(3):497-502. DOI: 10.3892/or.13.3.497

[4] Hishida I, Nanba H, Kuroda H. Mint: Antitumor activity exhibited by orally administered extract from fruit body of Grifola frondosa (maitake). Chemical & Pharmaceutical Bulletin. 1988;**36**(5): 1819-1827. DOI: 10.1248/cpb.36.1819

[5] Mayell M. Maitake extracts and their therapeutic potential. Alternative Medicine Review. 2001;**6**(1):48-60

[6] Abdullaev FI. Plant-derived agents against cancer. In: Gupta SK, editor. Pharmacology and Therapeutics in the New Millennium. New Delhi: Narosa Publishing House; 2001. pp. 345-354. ISBN: 0792370597

[7] Kodama N, Komuta K, Nanba H. Mint: Effect of Maitake (Grifola frondosa) D-fraction on the activation of NK cells in cancer patients. Journal of Medicinal Food. 2003;**6**(4):371-377. DOI: 10.1089/109662003772519949

[8] Kodama N, Komuta K, Sakai N, et al. Mint: Effects of D-fraction, a polysaccharide from Grifola frondosa on tumor growth involve activation of NK cells. Biological and Pharmaceutical Bulletin. 2002;**25**(12):1647-1650. DOI: 10.1248/bpb.25.1647

[9] Kodama N, Komuta K, Nanba H. Mint: Can maitake MD-fraction aid cancer patients? Alternative Medicine Review. 2002;**7**(3):236-239

[10] Nanba H, Kubo K. Mint: Effect of Maitake D-fraction on cancer prevention. Annals of the New York Academy of Sciences. 1997;**833**(1 Cancer):204-207. DOI: 10.1111/j.1749-6632.1997.tb48611.x

[11] Ferreira IC, Vaz JA, Vasconcelos MH, et al. Mint: Compounds from wild mushrooms with antitumor potential. Anti-Cancer Agents in Medicinal Chemistry. 2010; **10**(5):424-436. DOI: 10.2174/1871520611009050424

[12] De Silva DD, Rapior S, Fons F, et al. Mint: Medicinal mushrooms in supportive cancer therapies: An approach to anti-cancer effects and putative mechanisms of action. Fungal Diversity. 2012;**55**:1-35. DOI: 10.1007/s13225-012-0151-3

[13] Lull C, Wichers H, Savelkoul HF. Mint: Antiinflammatory and immunomodulating properties of fungal metabolites. Mediators of Inflammation. 2005;(2):63-68. DOI: 10.1155/MI.2005.63

[14] Chen J, Seviour R. Mint: Medicinal importance of fungal β–(1,3), (1,6)-glucans. Rev. Mycological Research. 2007;**111**(Pt. 6):635-652. DOI: 10.1016/j.mycres.2007.02.011

[15] Abbas AK, Lichtman AH, Pillai S. Inmunología Celular y Molecular. 6th ed. Barcelona, España: Elsevier Science Publishers; 2010. ISBN: 9788491133773

[16] Chi-Fung Chan G, Keung Chan W, Man-Yuen Sze D. Mint: The effects of β-glucan on human immune and cancer cells. Journal of Hematology & Oncology. 2009;**2**:25. DOI: 10.1186/1756-8722-2-25

[17] Masuda Y, Togo T, Mizuno S, et al. Mint: Soluble beta-glucan from Grifola frondosa induces proliferation and Dectin-1/Syk signaling in resident macrophages via the GM-CSF autocrine pathway. Journal of Leukocyte Biology. 2012;**91**(4):547-556. DOI: 10.1189/jlb.0711386

[18] Kodama N, Yamada M, Nanba H. Mint: Addition of Maitake D-fraction reduces the effective dosage of vancomycin for the treatment of listeria-infected mice. Japanese Journal of Pharmacology. 2001;**87**(4):327-332. DOI: 10.1254/jjp.87.327

[19] Inoue A, Kodama N, Nanba H. Mint: Effect of maitake (Grifola frondosa) D-fraction on the control of the T lymph node Th-1/Th-2 proportion. Biological & Pharmaceutical Bulletin. 2002;**25**(4): 536-540. DOI: 10.1248/bpb.25.536

[20] Sanzen I, Imanishi N, Takamatsu N, et al. Mint: Nitric oxide mediated antitumor activity induced by the extract from Grifola frondosa (Maitake mushroom) in a macrophage cell line, RAW264.7. Journal of Experimental & Clinical Cancer Research. 2001;**20**(4): 591-597

[21] Svagelj M, Berovic M, Gregori A, et al. Mint: Immunomodulating activities of cultivated maitake medicinal mushroom Grifola frondosa (dicks.: Fr.) S.F. gray (higher basidiomycetes) on peripheral blood mononuclear cells. International Journal of Medicinal Mushrooms. 2012;**14**(4): 377-383. DOI: 10.1615/IntJMedMushr.v14.i4.50

[22] Masuda Y, Murata Y, Hayashi M, et al. Mint: Inhibitory effect of MD-fraction on tumor metastasis: Involvement of NK cell activation and suppression of intercellular adhesion molecule (ICAM)-1 expression in lung vascular endothelial cells. Biological & Pharmaceutical Bulletin. 2008;**31**(6): 1104-1108. DOI: 10.1248/bpb.31.1104

[23] Harada N, Kodama N, Nanba H. Mint: Relationship between dendritic cells and the D-fraction-inducedTh-1 dominant response in BALB/c tumor-bearing mice. Cancer Letters. 2003; **192**(2):181-187. DOI: 10.1016/s0304-3835(02)00716-4

[24] Baran J, Allendorf DJ, Hong F, et al. Mint: Oral β-glucan adjuvant therapy converts nonprotective Th2 response to protective Th1 cell-mediated immune response in mammary tumor-bearing mice. Folia Histochemica et Cytobiologica. 2007;**45**(2):107-114. DOI: 10.5603/4540.

[25] Yang TY, Yi W, Wen J, et al. Mint: Therapeutic effect of Jin long capsule combined with neoadjuvant chemotherapy on invasive breast cancer and the expression change of multidrug resistance proteins. Zhonghua Zhong Liu Za Zhi. 2019;**41**(2):118-123. DOI: 10.3760/cma.j.issn.0253-3766.2019.02.008

[26] Fesel PH, Zuccaro A. β-Glucan: Crucial component of the fungal cell wall and elusive MAMP in plants. Fungal Genetics and Biology. 2016;**90**: 53-60. DOI: 10.1016/j.fgb.2015.12.004

[27] Büchele Rodrigues E, Penha FM, Melo GM, et al. CHAPTER 15 - Retina and ocular toxicity to ocular application of drugs. In: Retinal Pharmacotherapy. São Paulo, Brazil: Elsevier; 2010. pp. 96-103. DOI: 10.1016/B978-1-4377-0603-1.00020-X

[28] Giles AJ, Hutchinson MKND, Sonnemann HM, et al. Dexamethasone-induced immunosuppression: Mechanisms and implications for immunotherapy. Journal for Immuno

Therapy of Cancer. 2018;**6**:51. DOI: 10.1186/s40425-018-0371-5

[29] Liberman AC, Budziñski ML, Sokn C, et al. Regulatory and mechanistic actions of glucocorticoids on T and inflammatory cells. Frontiers in Endocrinology. 2018;**9**:235. DOI: 10.3389/fendo.2018.00235

[30] Wasser SP. Mint: Medicinal mushrooms science: History, current status, future trends and unsolved problems. International Journal of Medicinal Mushrooms. 2010;**12**(1):1-16. DOI: 10.1615/IntJMedMushr.v12.i1.10

[31] Pérez JE, Isaza G, Bueno JG, et al. Mint: Efecto de los extractos de Phenax rugosus, Tabebuia chrysantha, Althernantera williamsii y Solanum dolichosepalum sobre el leucograma y la producción de anticuerpos en ratas. Revista Medica de Risaralda. 2004; **10**(2):13-21. DOI: 10.22517/25395203.7953

[32] Kayser O, Masihi KN, Kiderlen AF. Mint: Natural products and synthetic compounds as immunomodulators. Expert Review of Anti-Infective Therapy. 2003;**1**(2):319-335. DOI: 10.1586/14787210.1.2.319

[33] Wasser SP, Didukh M, Nevo E. Mint: Antitumor and immunomodulatory activities of medicinal mushroom polysaccharide and polysaccharide-protein complexes in animals and humans (review). Mycologia Balcanica. 2005;**2**:221-250. DOI: 10.5281/zenodo.2547136

[34] Nakashima A, Yamada K, Iwata O, Sugimoto R, Atsuji K, Ogawa T, et al. βGlucan in foods and its physiological functions. Journal of Nutritional Science and Vitaminology. 2018;**64**(1):817

[35] Brown GD, Gordon S. Immune recognition. A new receptor for beta-glucans. Nature. 2001;**413**(6851):36-37

[36] Brown GD, Taylor PR, Reid DM, Willment JA, Williams DL, Martinez-Pomares L, et al. Dectin-1 is a major beta-glucan receptor on macrophages. The Journal of Experimental Medicine. 2002;**196**(3):407-412

[37] Hong F, Yan J, Baran JT, Allendorf DJ, Hansen RD, Ostroff GR, et al. Mechanism by which orally administered beta-1,3-glucans enhance the tumoricidal activity of antitumor monoclonal antibodies in murine tumor models. Journal of Immunology. 2004; **173**(2):797-806

[38] Niu L, Chen Q, Hua C, et al. Mint: Effects of chronic dexamethasone administration on hyperglycemia and insulin release in goats. Journal of Animal Science and Biotechnology. 2018;**9**:26. DOI: 10.1186/s40104-018-0242-4

[39] Estrada A, van Kessel A, Laarveld B. Mint: Effect of administration of oat beta-glucan on immune parameters of healthy and immunosuppressed beef steers. Canadian Journal of Veterinary Research. 1999;**63**(4):261-268

[40] Kotthoff P, Heine A, Held SAE, et al. Mint: Dexamethasone induced inhibition of Dectin-1 activation of antigen presenting cells is mediated via STAT-3 and NF-κB signaling pathways. Scientific Reports. 2017;7(1):4522. DOI: 10.1038/s41598-017-04558-z

[41] Masuda Y, Inoue H, Ohta H, et al. Mint: Oral administration of soluble β-glucans extracted from Grifola frondosa induces systemic antitumor immune response and decreases immunosuppression in tumor-bearing mice. International Journal of Cancer. 2013;**133**(1):108-119. DOI: 10.1002/ijc.27999

[42] Lin H, De Stanchina E, Zhou XK, et al. Mint: Maitake beta-glucan enhances umbilical cord blood stem cell transplantation in the NOD/SCID

mouse. Experimental Biology and Medicine. 2009;**234**(3):342-353. DOI: 10.3181/0807-RM-226

[43] Kodama N, Murata Y, Asakawa A, et al. Mint: Maitake D-fraction enhances antitumor effects and reduces immunosuppression by mitomycin-C in tumor-bearing mice. Nutrition. 2005; **21**(5):624-629. DOI: 10.1016/j.nut.2004.09.021

[44] Kay J, Czop JK. Enhancement of human monocyte beta-glucan receptors by glucocorticoids. Immunology. 1994; **81**(1):96-102

Chapter 6

The Role of Mushrooms in Biodegradation and Decolorization of Dyes

Abu Barkat Md Gulzar, Udaya Kumar Vandana, Prosenjit Paul and Pranab B. Mazumder

Abstract

Contamination of soil, water, and air by hazardous substances is the major environmental problem of today's world. Mushroom consumption has become a tradition among many people due to its richness in flavors, proteins, and some medicinal importance. But its ability to degrade/decolorize hazardous substances and dyes by secreting various enzymes or by absorption and adsorption of colors from waste substances has made them of interest for use in the field of bioremediation. Mushroom acts as a good decomposer as it degrades cellulose and lignin of plants for their growth and development. It also maintains soil health by performing the role of hyperaccumulators. This chapter focused on the mushroom-based biodegradation/decolorization of dyes and effluents released from various industries or other sources. It also emphasizes the probable mechanisms involved in mushroom-based degradation and decolorization of dyes along with their recent achievements, advancements, and future prospective.

Keywords: mushroom, biodegradation, biosorption, bioconversion, decolorization, dye, agro-industrial wastes

1. Introduction

To fulfill the demand of growing number of people, rapid industrialization and modernization not only give useful products but also release hazardous elements to nature. The release of industrial effluents and the accumulation of toxic substances into the biosphere destroy the environment by interacting with various components of the natural ecosystem [1]. The effluents released from textile industries, food processing industries, pharmaceutical industries, etc., containing various synthetic dyes, toxic heavy metals, and other wastes, directly or indirectly come in contact with water and soil and destroy water and soil properties by changing the pH, total organic carbon (TOC), biological oxygen demand (BOD), and chemical oxygen demand (COD) [1, 2]. Various types of synthetic dyes are used extensively in the field of textile industries for coloring purposes. For example in batik industries, Remazol Brilliant Blue R (RBBR) and naphthol are used as coloring agents. Remazol Brilliant Blue R is a heterocyclic compound, and its derivatives are toxic to the environment. On the other hand, naphthol is insoluble in water and is used to dye cellulosic fibers. Improper handling, carelessness, and inefficient dye waste treatments of industries are the main reasons for the contamination of soil and water [3]. The concentration of carcinogenic heavy metals like As, Cd, Co, Cr, Cu, Fe, Hg, Mn, Ni, etc. are relatively high in untreated industrial wastes. The rapid depletion of dissolved oxygen in water due to the presence of toxic heavy metals and other industrial wastes leads to "oxygen sag" [1]. Majority of the synthetic dyes are used in the field of textile industries, and the effluents are discharged as wastewater. The dyes or their breakdown products are hazardous they are found to be carcinogenic [4].

Remediation refers to the complete or partial removal of contaminants from the polluted sites to provide a sustainable environment. Various physical and chemical remediation technologies are developed to eliminate the pollutant from the soil and improve soil health. Higher costs, limited applications with limited opportunities, and the inability to enhance intrinsic soil health make them almost abandoned [5]. Bioremediation refers to the use of biological agents such as microbes, plants, or any other living things that help to reduce contamination to a nontoxic level or untraceable level [5]. Paul Stamets first coined the term "mycoremediation" based on the fungal detoxification of contaminated soil. He defined the term mycoremediation as a process of sequestration of contaminated soil or water by using fungi to reduce contaminants [6]. Mushrooms are sources of protein and their enzymatic machinery have the ability to degrade pollutants for their growth and developments. Thus, mushroom cultivation got much more attention in the field of decolorization and biodegradation research. Mushrooms are mostly basidiomycetes, a class of fungi which secretes a variety of extracellular enzymes for their growth and development [7]. These enzymes include laccase, lignin peroxidase (LiP), versatile peroxidase (VP), manganese peroxidase (MnP), phenoloxidases, etc. [8]. Singh reported that the lignin degradation ability of white-rot fungi is due to the presence of phenoloxidase [1]. Due to the potential role in bioremediation of various dyes, lignin, and cellulosic compounds, the white-rot fungi became a model organism for mycoremediation [1]. Due to the structural similarity of polycyclic aromatic hydrocarbons (PAH), polychlorinated biphenyl (PCB), various dyes, dioxins, and pesticides with lignin, cellulosic compounds, and with their substrates, mushroom-based mycoremediation processes got much more emphasized in the recent years [9]. This chapter focused on the mushroom-based biodegradation/decolorization of dyes and effluents released from various industries or other sources. It also emphasizes the probable mechanisms involved in mushroom-based degradation and decolorization of dyes along with their recent achievements, advancements, and future prospective.

2. Role of mushroom in decolorization of dyes

Industries like textile, food processing, chemical, leather, dyestuff, dyeing, and pharmaceutical industries release a huge number of effluents containing various types of dyes. Textile industries are thought to be leading producers of dyes, and the dyes released from industries directly penetrate into the soil and water and disturb the natural ecosystem [10]. Around 80,000 tons of dyestuff and shades are created in India. It has been assessed that 10,000 distinctive colored materials are economically accessible worldwide and the yearly generation is evaluated to be 7×10^5 metric tons [11]. In the field of textile industries, azo dyes are mostly used as a colorant agent. The presence of one or more azo groups helps to prevent the molecules from breakdown and degradation and hence persistently accumulated into the environment. The entry of industrial effluents into the water causes a drastic reduction of dissolved oxygen; as a result great environmental damage will occur [10]. The entry of dyes into the aquatic ecosystem disturbs light penetration into the deeper part; as a result, reduction of water quality, photosynthetic activity, as well as gas availability into the aquatic ecosystem is observed [6].

Different physical and chemical methods are developed for decolorization of dyes from the pollutant sites which includes absorption through activated carbon, flocculation, ion exchange, membrane filtration, etc. but due to high expensive, inefficient, and these methods also release different types of wastes which are also toxic for nature [10]. On the other hand, mushroom-based decolorization and degradation of dyes got much more research attention because it is less expensive and eco-friendly and also produces negligible amounts of wastes [6]. Due to the powerful enzymatic activities as well as high adaptability under physically harsh conditions, microbial decolorization and biodegradation is one of the most focused research areas for sustainable developments [1]. Aromatic amines, phenolics, etc. are some intermediates generated during decolorization processes which are highly toxic with low biodegradability as compared to dye. Sometimes, such intermediates inhibit the decolorization ability of bacteria. While fungi have the ability to degrade complex organic compounds and the intermediates through their extracellular enzymes secretion. On the other hand, it is thought that the large surface area of fungi has a greater ability for biodegradation [12]. The decolorization ability of dyes varies from strain to strain, and most of the studies are confined to single-strain-based degradation or decolorization of specific dyes. However, industrial effluents are a cocktail of various organic and inorganic pollutants. Considering these factors, the researcher proposed that the use of novel microbial consortium in the field of bioremediation could be a better option [13]. And many reports suggest that the microbial consortium possesses greater biodegradation ability due to their interactive effect with the contaminants [13–15]. According to Forgacs et al., the individual strain of a consortium has a specialized role for specific contaminants and may attack the different portions of dye and also has the ability to degrade the intermediate components such as phenolics and aromatic hydrocarbons produced by co-strains [16]. By using this approach, several components of the contaminants can be treated at the same time.

Biodegradation and decolorization ability of mushroom has shown a promising approach since the 1980s. There are many reports regarding the decolorization of different types of dyes by using mushrooms. Cripps et al. reported the decolorization of azo dyes by ligninolytic enzymes secreted by *Phanerochaete chrysosporium*, a white-rot fungus [17]. A similar degrading activity was later reported on another species of white-rot fungi [18]. White-rot fungi have a variety of advantages that can be utilized in the field of bioremediation. The extracellular lignin-degrading system of white-rot fungi has the ability to degrade various toxic chemicals like polyhydroxy aromatic carbons and other phenolic compounds [19]. Freitag and Morrell screened 170 fungal strains to understand the decolorization of poly R-478, a polymeric dye, through ligninolytic activity of the fungi and the existence of peroxidase and phenoloxidase activity. In the plate test, they found that the decolorization rate increased with the increase of radial growth of fungi, indicating that decolorization is directly correlated with hyphal development [20]. Reddy et al. reported that the growth of white-rot fungi through hyphal extension and hence penetration of fungal hyphae into the contaminated soil could help in bioremediation [12, 20]. While, according to Moreno-Garrido, immobilization of mushroom fungi is one of the strategies for biodegradation [21]. Yao et al. studied the decolorization of three different azo dyes by extracellular enzymes produced by *Schizophyllum* sp. F17, and they found that manganese peroxidase (MnP) played an important role in the process of decolorization [22]. The copper-containing laccase is one of the important enzymes that also play a significant role in the bioremediation of dyes. Lallawmsanga et al. screened 40 enzymes for their laccase productions and their role in decolorization of dyes. They found eight strains that have elevated levels of laccase producing ability; *P. pulmonarius* BPSM10 strain decolorizes seven dyes under the aqueous condition and can be used as an alternative biosorbent to decolorize dyes under aqueous condition [23]. Chakraborty et al. reported another white-rot fungus *Alternaria alternata* CMERI F6 having a 99.99% decolorization ability of Congo red within 48 h. The metabolites produced through HPLC and FTIR suggested that the decolorization of dye occurred through the biosorption and biodegradation process [24]. Mahmoud in 2016 studied the decolorization ability of Baker's yeast under aqueous condition. He reported that Baker's yeast can reduce the color and COD of textile effluents by 100% and 61.8% and can be used for bioremediation [25]. Another white-rot fungal strain, KRUS-G, is able to decolorize Remazol Brilliant Blue R up to 1500 ppm concentration by secreting laccase and manganese peroxidase. And it is also reported that an increase in concentration slightly decreases the hyphal growth [26].

3. Mechanism of mushroom-based decolorization of dyes

The biodegradation or decolorization of dyes mainly consists of three basic processes [1, 27]. These are as follows:

1. A slight change in additional organic molecules without changing the main structure of the compounds.

2. Fractionation of the complex structural organic molecules in such a way that the combination of the fractions could give rise to the original molecules.

3. Mineralization of the complex structural molecules, i.e., transformation of the complex molecules into the mineral forms.

It is thought that adsorption of the dyes is the primary mechanism of dye decolorization by fungus or any other biological mode of decolorization. In many reports, it was found that adsorption of dyes is the important mechanism of dye decolorization by which the transformation of dyes starts [1, 28]. Microscopic observation of the fungal cells showed that instead of fungal hyphae, fungal spores are the main dye-absorbing components [1]. Hydrophilic and hydrophobic interactions of fungi and dyestuff play a crucial role in the enhancement of dye absorption [28]. Some reports also state that when the concentration of extracellular enzymes and cell mass increased, the dye color in the medium decreased indicating that the decolorization of dyestuff is directly proportional to the cell mass as well as the extracellular enzymes produced by the fungus [1].

Mushroom-based degradation or decolorization of dyes is mainly classified into [1] biosorption and [2] biodegradation [1, 29].

3.1 Bio-sorption

Biosorption is a complex physicochemical method of biological materials that have the ability to accumulate pollutants into cellular components through adsorption, ion exchange, deposition, etc. and plays an important role in dye decolorization by fungi [1, 30]. Fu and Viraraghavan reported that the decolorization of dyes like Disperse Red I, Congo red, Acid Blue 29, and Basic Blue 9 by *Aspergillus niger* is due to the presence of carboxyl, amino phosphate group, and lipid fractions [31].

Carboxyl, amino phosphate group, and lipid fractions together act as a binding site for Congo red. While for decolorization of Basic Blue 9, carboxyls, and amino groups are the binding sides. The amino group of *Aspergillus niger* alone acts as a binding site for Acid Blue 29, whereas amino groups along with lipid fractions have the binding ability for Disperse Red I. They also reported that along with adsorption, electrostatic attraction mechanisms also have a crucial role in dye decolorization [9].

Fu and Viraraghavan from their study suggested that the adsorption efficiency could be enhanced by treating the biomass with suitable organic or inorganic molecules like formaldehyde, sulfuric acid, sodium hydroxide, calcium chloride, and sodium bicarbonate and by high temperature. Increase in temperature by autoclaving and chemical treatments by 0.1 N NaOH, 0.1 M HCl, and 0.1 M H_2SO_4 increased the biosorption. It was found that the physical treatments increased the biosorption rate of the Basic Blue 9 dye by 15 times, whereas chemical treatment with 0.1 M H_2SO_4 enhanced the rate of biosorption of Acid Blue 29 dye by 2 times. The physical treatment of autoclaving of fungal biomass could change the surface charge, and acid pretreatment enhanced the affinity of anionic dyes to bind with the fungal surface [31]. Arica and Bayramoğlu also observe the same result by autoclaving *Lentinus sajor-caju* at 100°C for 10 min; the biosorption capacity of fungal biomass *Lentinus sajor-cafju* for Reactive Red 120 dye increased [32]. A number of a research articles have been published based on the dye biosorption ability of mushroom fungi, and these are depicted in **Table 1**.

Serial number	Mushroom used	Name of the dye	Remarks	References
1.	*Ganoderma* sp.	Orange II, 10B (Blue), RS (Red)	*Ganoderma* sp. able to degrade woods, based on this fact the decolorization test against those dyes showed significant results	[33]
2.	*Agaricus bisporus*	*Basic Red 18*, Levafix Braun E-RN, Acid Red 111	Mushroom stump wastes are found to play a promising role in the decolorization of wastewater containing dyes released from various industries. Freeze-dried mushroom stumps showed higher decolorization efficiency for basic dyes, while heat-dried stumps showed greater biosorption efficiency for acidic dyes	[34]
3.	*Pleurotus ostreatus*	Malachite green, xylidine	pH plays an important role in dye decolorization. Maximum biosorption was observed at pH 3 for malachite green, while, for xylidine, the pH values varied from pH 3 to 4	[35]
4.	*Pleurotus ostreatus*	Malachite green	Biosorbant dose, time, and pH were important factors for biosorption. Ca^+ and Na^+ ions play a crucial role in biosorption. The presence of hydroxyl, carboxylic acid, phosphate, and amino group on the surface of biosorbent, i.e., *Pleurotus ostreatus*, was confirmed by FTIR	[36]
5.	*Lentinus sajor-caju*	Reactive Red 120	Maximum uptake was noticed at pH 3.0 for all the fungal preparations. And highest dye uptake efficiencies were observed in heat-treated preparations followed by acid-treated, native, and base-treated preparations	[32]

Serial number	Mushroom used	Name of the dye	Remarks	References
6.	*Agaricus bisporus* and *Thuja orientalis*	Reactive Blue 49 (RB49)	Mix culture of *Agaricus bisporus* and *Thuja orientalis* showed efficient decolorization of Reactive Blue 49 (RB49) dye by biosorption. FTIR and SEM analysis confirmed the presence of hydroxyl, carboxyl, amine, and amide groups on the surface of biosorbent	[37]
7.	*Pleurotus ostreatus*	Methylene Blue	The biosorption ability of a white-rot fungi *Pleurotus ostreatus* is studied against Methylene Blue. And it was found that pH, dye concentration, and fungal biomass plays an essential role in biosorption	[37]
8.	*Agaricus bisporus*	Crystal Violet-Brilliant Green	Thermodynamic studies show that Crystal Violet-Brilliant Green adsorption by *Agaricus bisporus* is a spontaneous process. Dye-fungus interaction was studied by SEM, X-ray crystallography, and Fourier transform electron spectroscopy to understand the mechanism of dye adsorption. And it was concluded that the process is eco-friendly and economical and can be used for the cationic dye biosorption process	[38]
9.	*Agaricus bisporus* and *Thuja orientalis*	Reactive Red 45	Biosorption of Reactive Red 45 by *Agaricus bisporus* and *Thuja orientalis* is highly pH-dependent, and the process is spontaneous and exothermic. Mix culture treatment showed 100% biosorption. It can be used as an alternative mode of biosorbent for industrial dye removal	[39]
10.	*Lentinus concinnus*	Disperse Red 60	Immobilized fungal biomass of *Lentinus concinnus* has maximum biosorption at pH 6.0 and can be used for Disperse Red 60 dye removal from industrial effluents	[40]

Table 1.
Role of mushrooms in biosorption of dyes.

3.2 Biodegradation

Biodegradation is the process by which complex organic molecules are converted into its simpler forms by the action of enzymes secreted by fungi, bacteria, or any other living microorganisms [41]. A lot of studies have been carried out to understand dye degradation by mushrooms and the enzyme produced by them, and these are represented in **Table 2**. Many reports suggested that the extracellular enzymes produced by mushroom have a potential role in dye decolorization and also have degradability for non-polymeric compounds like polyhydroxy aromatic hydrocarbons, nitrotoluene, and pentachlorophenol under in vitro conditions [46]. In recent years, degradation of polymeric compounds like plastics by various types of mushrooms is also reported [51].

Serial number	Mushroom used	Name of the dye	Enzyme produced	References
1.	*Pleurotus pulmonarius BPSM10*	Malachite green	Laccase	[23]
2.	*Pleurotus ostreatus*	Remazol Brilliant Blue R	Manganese peroxidase, manganese-independent peroxidase, and phenoloxidase	[42]
3.	*P. ostreatus*, *P. sapidus*, *P. florida*	Coralene Golden Yellow, Coralene Navy Blue, and Coralene Dark Red	Laccase, manganese-dependent peroxidase (MnP), and lignin peroxidase	[43]
4.	*Pleurotus pulmonarius*	Remazol Brilliant Blue R, Congo red, Methylene Blue, and ethyl violet	Laccase and manganese peroxidase	[44]
5.	*Pleurotus ostreatus*	Acetyl Yellow G (AYG), Remazol Brilliant Blue R or Acid Blue 129 (AB129)	Dye-decolorizing peroxidase (DyP)	[45]
6.	*Lentinus edodes*	Poly-478 and Remazol Brilliant Blue R	Manganese peroxidase	[1]
7.	*Lasiodiplodia* sp.	Malachite green	Laccases	[46]
8.	*Pleurotus ostreatus*	Synthetic dye	Laccases, lignin peroxidases	[47]
9.	*Pleurotus florida*	Blue CA, Black B133, Corazol Violet SR	Laccases	[48]
10.	*Pleurotus pulmonarius*	CK, Congo red, Trypan blue, methyl green, Remazol Brilliant Blue R (RBB), methyl violet, ethyl violet, and Brilliant Cresyl Blue	Laccases	[29]
11.	*Ganoderma* sp.	Textile effluents	Laccases	[49]
12.	*Pleurotus ostreatus IBL-02*	Synthetic dye	Ligninolytic enzymes	[50]

Table 2.
Role of mushroom in biodegradation of dyes by means of enzymatic secretions.

The degradation of polycyclic aromatic carbons by cleaving a carbon-carbon single bond is an important feature of white-rot fungi [1]. The lignin-degrading enzymes of white-rot fungi such as lignin peroxidases or ligninases have a potential role to initiate oxidative depolymerization of lignin for degradation of various organo-pollutants. The ligninolytic activity of a white-rot fungi *P. chrysosporium* has the capability to degrade various industrial dyes and other toxic aromatic ring-containing compounds [52]. Various mechanisms have recently been identified for fungi-based degradation of dyes. The generation of free radicals by white-rot fungi for the degradation of various synthetic dyes or other pollutants is one of the best-known mechanisms or decolorization of dyes [1]. Due to their highly reactive nature, free radicals are able to donate or accept electrons from other chemicals, and sometimes chain reactions occur due

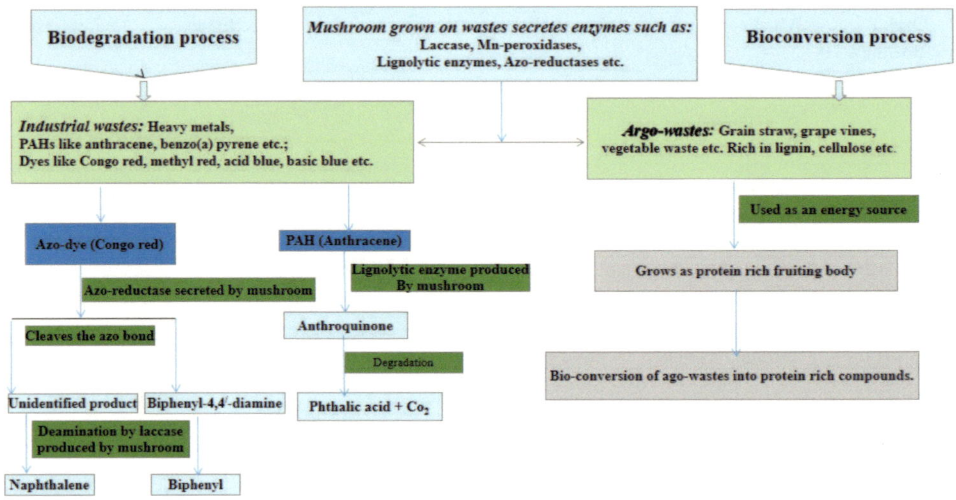

Figure 1.
Schematic representation of mushroom-based enzymatic biodegradation and bioconversion of dyes and other agro-wastes.

to donation and accepting of electrons, and also various radicals are generated along with the formation of initial radicals. These free radicals are catalyzed by peroxidase enzymes produced by white-rot fungi which play a subsequent role in the degradation process of various industrial pollutants [1, 53, 54]. The role of veratryl alcohol in azo dye degradation catalyzed by ligninase enzyme produced by white-rot fungi along with H_2O_2 was reported by Paszczynski and Crawford [55]. Peroxidases, laccases, and azoreductases are the major enzymes produced by mushrooms during the biodegradation of dyes. Azo linkage and chromophoric groups of azo dyes are reduced by the enzyme azoreductases produced by mushrooms responsible for azo dye degradation (**Figure 1**) [56]. An edible mushroom *Lentinus edodes* which produces a high amount of manganese peroxidase degrade Poly-478 and Remazol Brilliant Blue R [1]. Vyas and Molitoris reported the decolorization of Brilliant Blue R by mushroom *Pleurotus ostreatus* by secreting H_2O_2-dependent enzymes [42]. Laccase enzyme produced by *P. pulmonarius* BPSM10 showed efficient dye decolorization, especially malachite green (MG). The decolorization efficiency of *P. pulmonarius* BPSM10 was confirmed by FTIR [23].

4. Degradation of agricultural pesticides, chemical, and other wastes

Nowadays, agricultural management practices depend on the efficient management of biotic factors such as insects, pests, various diseases, weeds, etc.; otherwise, plant growth and development along with crop yields would decrease drastically. To minimize such drastic loss in crop production, there is continuous use of insecticides, pesticides, weedicides, and chemical fertilizers constantly releasing xenobiotic compounds into the environments [19, 57]. Xenobiotic compounds are not easily degraded by microbes and hence remain active in the soil and water [58]. The use of pesticides in India is considerably increasing after 2009–2010. It was reported that the consumption of pesticides in 2014–2015 is 0.29 kg/ha which is 50% higher than that in 2019–2010 [59]. According to previous reports, only 5% of the applied pesticides are effective in targeted pest management, and the rest of the pesticides are mixed with soil and water, affecting human health by interfering with the food chain [60, 61]. On the other hand, modernization, industrialization, and other anthropogenic activities continuously releasing wastes containing hazardous compounds like heavy metals, dyes, phenolic compounds, polyhydroxy aromatic hydrocarbons, etc. are also disturbing agricultural lands [19].

5. The mechanism involved in the degradation of agrochemicals and other wastes by mushroom

Mushroom-based degradation of agrochemical wastes, heavy metals, phenolics, polyhydroxy aromatic hydrocarbons, and other wastes basically involves enzymatic degradation, biosorption, and bioconversion techniques. Researchers have published a number of research articles on mushroom-based biodegradation of agronomic wastes [19, 62].

5.1. Enzymatic degradation of agricultural wastes

Mycologists and environmental researchers are giving attention to enzymatic degradation of agricultural wastes by using mushrooms. However, the proper role of enzymes in pesticide degradation is not clear. But there is some evidence suggesting that lignin-degrading enzymes are responsible for pesticide degradation. Mushrooms do not secrete pesticide-degrading enzymes in a similar manner; that is, it varies from species to species, type of condition, and other physical and chemical factors [5, 19]. Xenobiotics are chemical compounds that are found in the environment but not naturally produced in the environments. Sometimes, a naturally occurring component is also called xenobiotic when it is excessively available in the environment. Xenobiotics are not easily degradable in nature and hence actively present into the environment. Polycyclic aromatic hydrocarbons, alkanes, oil spills, azo dyes, antibiotics, dioxins, polychlorinated, chlorinated, polyaromatic compounds, etc. are major xenobiotics continuously released into the environment [63]. Microbes play a significant role in the field of biodegradation. There are some reports suggesting the involvement of mushroom fungi in the degradation process of agrochemicals such as xenobiotics, heavy metals, and other agricultural wastes by secreting various enzymes like oxidoreductases, laccases, oxygenase, and peroxidases. These enzymes can degrade the hazardous compounds by the breakdown of ester, amide, ether bonds, and sometimes the aromatic ring or the aliphatic chains of those compounds [6, 19, 64]. The concentration of hazardous compounds, reaction conditions, and the suitable sites are also responsible for the degradation of such compounds. Sometimes, xenobiotic compounds are utilized by mushrooms for their growth and development as their source of energy, carbon, nitrogen, and sulfur [6]. Some researchers reported that the ligninolytic enzyme produced by mushrooms can degrade the PAHs into mineral forms. For example, the ligninolytic enzyme produced by *P. chrysosporium* can produce anthraquinone by degrading anthracene, a PAH. Further degradation of anthraquinone can produce phthalic acid and carbon dioxide (**Figure 1**) [65]. Few examples of mushroom which have the ability to degrade agrochemical pollutants by secreting enzymes are listed in **Table 3**.

As there are so many reports on enzymatic degradation of xenobiotics, there are also some reports on the non-ligninolytic degradation of xenobiotics. Jackson et al. reported the degradation of 2,4,6-Trinitrotoluene (TNT) by *P. chrysosporium* in the absence of ligninolytic enzymes [80]. Bending et al. also reported white-rot fungal degradation of atrazine and terbuthylazine in the aqueous condition in the absence of ligninolytic enzymes [81].

Serial number	Mushroom used	Name of the pollutant	Enzyme produced	References
1.	*Pleurotus ostreatus*	Plastics	Lignocellulolytic enzymes	[66]
2.	*Lentinula edodes*	2,4-Dichlorophenol	Ligninolytic enzyme-derived vanillin	[67]
3.	*Pleurotus pulmonarius*	Radioactive cellulosic-based waste	Ligninolytic enzymes	[68]
4.	*Auricularia* sp., *Schizophyllum commune*, and *Polyporus* sp.	Malachite green	Biosorption and enzymatic degradation	[69]
5.	*Pleurotus pulmonarius*	Crude oil	Peroxidase	[70]
6.	*Coriolus versicolor*	PAHs	Laccase, manganese-dependent peroxidase, and lignin peroxidase	[71]
7.	*P. ostreatus*	Anthracene	Lignin peroxidase, laccase, and manganese peroxidase	[72]
8.	*Pleurotus ostreatus*	Green polyethylene	Laccase	[66]
9.	*Pleurotus palmonarius*, *Pleurotus tuber-regium*, *Lentinus squarrosulus*	Crude oil	Ligninolytic enzymes	[73]
10.	*Pleurotus tuber-regium*	Crude oil	Ligninolytic enzymes	[74]
11.	*Bjerkandera adusta*	PAHs, PCBs	lignin-degrading enzyme	[53]
12.	*Irpex lacteus*	PAHs, TNT, bisphenol, dimethyl, phthalate	Laccase, lignin peroxidase, manganese peroxidase, versatile peroxidase	[75]
13.	*Pleurotus ostreatus and Irpex lacteus*	PCBs	Oxidoreductases	[76]
14.	*Phanerochaete chrysosporium*	DDT, PHAs, PCBs,	Lip, MnP	[77]
15.	*Phanerochaete chrysosporium*	PAHs	Peroxidases (LiP, MnP)	[52]
16.	*Schizophyllum commune*, *Polyporus* sp.	Malachite green dye	Ligninolytic enzymes	[69]
17.	*Trametes versicolor*	Lignin, polycyclic aromatic hydrocarbons, polychlorinated biphenyl mixture, and a number of synthetic dyes	Ligninolytic enzymes	[75]
18.	*P. chrysosporium*	Styrene	Peroxidases	[78]
19.	*Pleurotus ostreatus* HP-1	Fluoranthene	Manganese peroxidase (MnP) and laccase	[79]

Table 3.
Role of mushrooms in degradation of pollutants by secreting enzymes.

Serial number	Mushroom species	Agro-industrial wastes	Results	References
1.	*V. volvacea*	Banana leaves	Improved yield and provide sustainable feed for ruminant animals	[83]
2.	*Lentinula edodes*	Wheat straw	Bioconversion of wheat straw by synthesizing lignocellulosic enzymes and increased yield.	[84]
3.	*Pleurotus sapidus*	Wheat straw, rice straw, corn stover, corncobs, sugarcane bagasse (SCB), and banana stalk (BS)	Bioconversion by producing ligninolytic and cellulolytic enzymes	[85]
4.	*Pleurotus tuber-regium*	Cotton waste, rice straw	Lipase, peroxidase, cellulase, carboxymethylcellulose enzyme activity increased	[86]
5.	*Pleurotus eous*, *Lentinus connatus*	Rice straw, banana stem, sorghum stalk	Yield increased, degradation of lignin was observed	[87]
6.	*Pleurotus florida*	Paper waste, cardboard industrial waste	High protein content was observed	[88]
7.	*Pleurotus ostreatus*	Sawdust	Temperature and pH are important factors for the growth of mushrooms	[89]
8.	*Volvariella volvacea*	Sawdust	Enzyme activity was measured, and high cellulosic activity is responsible for bioconversion	[90]
9.	*Pleurotus citrinopileatus*	Paper waste, cardboard waste	Basidiocarps are grown and having high nutrients with no genotoxicity	[91]
10.	*Pleurotus tuber-regium*	Rice straw, cocoyam peels	Yield improved with high protein content, fat content	[92]
11.	*Lentinula edodes*	Eucalyptus waste	Successful bioconversion by lignin degradation was observed. Qualitative and quantitative changes are also noticed	[93]
12.	*Lentinus tigrinus*	Wheat straw	Bioconversion of wheat straw and production of lignocellulosic enzymes are observed	[84]

Table 4.
Role of mushroom in bioconversion of agro-industrial wastes.

5.2 Bioconversion of agricultural wastes

Agro-industrial wastes are the by-products of agricultural processing industries such as grain milling industries, oilseed-processing industries, brewery industries, and fruit and vegetable processing industries. These agro-industrial wastes are rich in various nutrients and bioactive compounds. Nowadays, researchers employ attention in bioconversion of such agro-industrial wastes into some other useful components [5]. Mushroom cultivation on agro-industrial wastes is one of the most important examples of bioconversion where fruiting bodies are used as a product [82]. The choice of agro-industrial substrates depends upon the availability of the substrates [5]. Mushroom cultivated on agro-industrial wastes is mentioned in **Table 4**. As agro-industrial wastes are rich in nutrients, mushroom-based mycoremediation of such components gives rise to protein-rich fruiting bodies by degrading such industrial wastes (**Figure 1**) [82].

6. Biosorption of heavy metals

Biosorption is defined as "the ability of biologically active i.e. living or inactive i.e. non-living or dead organisms/materials that can accumulate and concentrate heavy metals even from very dilute medium by means of adsorption, absorption, ion-exchange or by using metabolic processes" [94]. Biosorption is a complex process, depending upon different factors like temperature, pH, the concentration of the substrates, nature of the substrates, contact time, as well as the property of the host, i.e., cell wall composition, types of proteins, amino acids, lipids, etc. [8, 19, 94].

In recent years, mushroom-based biosorption for waste management is one of the important research interests. A lot of research is going on regarding mushroom-based bioremediation for the cleanup of the environment, and mushroom-based biosorption of heavy metals is an important one [5]. Few reports on mushroom-based biosorptions of heavy metals are mentioned in **Table 5**.

Serial number	Mushroom species	Pollutants	Results	References
1.	*Pleurotus sajor-caju*	Heavy metals	Absorb heavy metals from contaminated sites	[95]
2.	*Pleurotus ostreatus*	Cadmium	Mushrooms are grown on the substrate containing cadmium and absorbed cadmium by the fruiting bodies	[96]
3.	*Pleurotus tuber-regium*	Heavy metals	Mushroom species are grown in soil by mixing heavy metals and played an efficient role in bioabsorption	[97]
4.	*Flammulina velutipes*	Copper	*Flammulina velutipes* were grown in aqueous conditions containing copper and were found as an efficient bioabsorbant	[98]
5.	*Pleurotus platypus*, *Agaricus bisporus*, *Calocybe indica*	Copper, zinc, iron, cadmium, lead, nickel	Mushroom species are grown in aqueous wastes containing heavy metals (copper, zinc, iron, cadmium, lead, and nickel and were found as an efficient bioabsorbant	[99]
6.	*Fomes fasciatus*	Copper	Mushroom species showed efficient bioabsorption of copper	[100]
7.	*Agaricus bisporus*, *Lactarius piperatu*	Cadmium	*Agaricus bisporus*, Lactarius piperatu has higher cadmium removal efficiency	[101]

Table 5.
Role of mushroom in bioremediation of heavy metal pollutants by biosorption process.

7. Factors affecting the degradation

Biodegradation by means of mushroom basically depends on the survival and multiplication of mushrooms [102]. Different intrinsic and extrinsic factors play an essential role in mushroom survival and multiplication. Substrate concentration, source of nitrogen, carbon-nitrogen ratio, pH, moisture, minerals, particle size, spawning level, surfactant, etc. are important intrinsic factors, while temperature, humidity, luminosity, air composition, etc. are extrinsic factors [103]. Alteration on those factors largely affects mushroom multiplications, and ultimately mushrooms will be unable to survive [102, 103].

pH plays an essential role in mushroom growth and it varies from mushroom to mushroom. Bellettini et al. reported the pH value of 4.0–7.0 helps mycelium growth, while pH value between 6.5 and 7.0 helps basidiocarp development [103]. Velioglu and Ozturk Urek reported that pH of 6.0 gives better growth of *P. djamor* [104].

Moisture is another important factor for mushroom growth as the flow of moisture helps to transfer nutrients from mycelium to fruiting body [105]. High moisture contents cause difficulties for mycelium respiration and interpretation of the development of the fruiting body, while low moisture contents lead to the death of the fruiting body [103]. Chang and Miles reported that 50–75% of moisture contents are suitable for the growth of mushrooms [105].

8. Advantages of mushroom-based mycoremediation

Mushroom cultivation under suitable conditions can help to detoxify various types of contaminants by secreting different types of nonspecific enzymes [106]. Hyphae help to establish direct contact with the contaminants [95]. Mushroom-based bioremediation of pollutants have several advantages, which are mentioned below:

- Due to the low cost, it got much more public acceptance.
- Safe and eco-friendly technique.
- Easy and simple cultivation process.
- Low maintenance.
- Mushrooms grow faster and produce reusable end products.

9. Limitations of mushroom-based degradation

The role of mushrooms in bioremediation of environmental pollutants like industrial wastes containing dyes; heavy metals; agrochemical wastes like pesticides, herbicides, insecticides, and other xenobiotic compounds; and agro-industrial wastes like brewery wastes, grain milling wastes, and fruits and vegetable processing wastes are studied [85]. However, certain drawbacks are noticed in mushroom-based remediation. Fungi-based degradation of pesticides is a slower and incomplete process; accumulation of incomplete substrate produces various secondary metabolites that might be harmful [19]. Adaptation of the chosen mushroom species against the pollutant is another major problem of mushroom-based bioremediation [5]. Physicochemical properties of soil and climatic conditions are sometimes problematic for bulk transfer of mushroom under field conditions [107]. The use of mushrooms with beneficial bacterial strain could help to degrade pollutants at faster rates. Identification of genes that are responsible for biodegradation of pollutants and the introduction of such genes to the indigenous strain could solve the availability of capable strain under field conditions [108]. Mushrooms are famous due to their richness in proteins and flavors and also for their medicinal importance. Mushrooms cultivated into the contaminated sites or cultivated for remediation of pollutants can accumulate different types of toxic substances into their fruiting bodies. Consumption of those mushrooms could cause major health problems and sometimes may become the reason for death [109].

10. Conclusion and future prospective

Logical advancements are considered as key components for the progression of underdeveloped countries. But the majority of industries do not have a legitimate waste treatment plan and discharge an enormous amount of effluents. The accomplishment of a microbial procedure for color removal from the industrial discharge relies upon the usage of microorganisms that viably decolorize manufactured colors of various compound structures. Most of the mushroom-based degradation/decolorization of dyes and other wastes has been performed under laboratory conditions. The outcomes gotten for the most part from the research facility tests rely upon explicit development and optimization of medium, proper handling of mushroom species, and biomass. Therefore, essential works on the topic are still under investigation to assess the information on the process of implementation under field conditions. Certain species of mushroom showed efficient degradation/decolorization/mineralization of the dyes, organochemicals, and other industrial wastes either by biosorption or by enzymatic secretion. Based on those facts, proper design of the waste management process by using proper strain is an essential step. The inhibition of growth and secretion of degrading enzymes of mushrooms by the contaminants containing different form of hazardous pollutants is another major problem in mushroom-based degradation of dyes or other pollutants. Utilizing molecular tools for identification of the genes responsible for the degradation of specific dyes may be helpful for biodegradation. Genetic engineering technologies for the development of genetically modified strain for the degradation or decolorization could solve the problem. The connection among the researchers of interdisciplinary research fields like biotechnology, microbiology, chemistry, and genetic engineering could help to develop a successful technique for bioremediations.

Author details

Abu Barkat Md Gulzar, Udaya Kumar Vandana, Prosenjit Paul and Pranab B. Mazumder*
Department of Biotechnology, Assam University, Silchar, India

*Address all correspondence to: uday21microb@gmail.com; pbmmmbl@gmail.com

References

[1] Singh L. Biodegradation of synthetic dyes: A mycoremediation approach for degradation/decolourization of textile dyes and effluents. Journal of Applied Biotechnology and Bioengineering. 2017;**3**(5):430-435

[2] Elango G, Rathika G, Elango S. Physico-chemical parameters of textile dyeing effluent and its impacts with case study. International Journal of Research in Chemistry and Environment. 2017;**7**(1):17-24

[3] Dewi RS, Ilyas M, Sari AA. Ligninolitic enzyme immobilization from *Pleurotus ostreatus* for dye and batik wastewater decolorization. Jurnal Pendidikan IPA Indonesia. 2019;**8**(2):220-229

[4] Gita S, Hussan A, Choudhury TG. Impact of textile dyes waste on aquatic environments and its treatment. Environment and Ecology. July 2017;**35**(3C):2349-2353

[5] Kulshreshtha S, Mathur N, Bhatnagar P. Mushroom as a product and their role in mycoremediation. AMB Express. 2014;**4**(1):1-7

[6] Chaudhary K, Agarwal S, Khan S. Role of phytochelatins (PCs), metallothioneins (MTs), and heavy metal ATPase (HMA) genes in heavy metal tolerance. In: Mycoremediation and Environmental Sustainability. Cham: Springer; 2018. pp. 39-60

[7] Elekes CC, Busuioc G. The mycoremediation of metals polluted soils using wild growing species of mushrooms. Latest trends on engineering education. Notulae Botanicae Horti Agrobotanici Cluj-Napoca. 22 July 2010;**38**:147-151

[8] Dutta SD, Hyder MD. Mycoremediation: A potential tool for sustainable management. Journal of Mycopathological Research. 2019;**57**(1):25-34

[9] Su K, Ka K, Lazur J. Biology of Macrofungi. 2018:129-157. Available from: http://link.springer.com/10.1007/978-3-030-02622-6

[10] Lalnunhlimi S, Veenagayathri K. Decolorization of azo dyes (Direct Blue 151 and Direct Red 31) by moderately alkaliphilic bacterial consortium. Brazilian Journal of Microbiology. 2016;**47**(1):39-46. DOI: 10.1016/j.bjm.2015.11.013

[11] Marimuthu T, Rajendran S, Manivannan M. A review on bacterial degradation of textile dyes. Journal of Chemistry and Chemical Sciences. 2013;**3**:201-212

[12] Reddy C. Symposium ZM-BMS, 2001 U. Bioremediation potential of white rot fungi. books.google.com [Internet]. 2001;**23**:52-78. Available from: https://books.google.co.in/books

[13] Mahapatra DM, Chanakya HN, Ramachandra TV. Bioremediation and lipid synthesis through mixotrophic algal consortia in municipal wastewater. Bioresource Technology. 2014;**168**:142-150

[14] Çetin D, Dönmez G. Decolorization of reactive dyes by mixed cultures isolated from textile effluent under anaerobic conditions. Enzyme and Microbial Technology. 2006;**38**(7):926-930

[15] Malaviya P, Rathore VS. Bioremediation of pulp and paper mill effluent by a novel fungal consortium isolated from polluted soil. Bioresource Technology. 2007;**98**(18):3647-3651

[16] Forgacs E, Cserháti T, Oros G. Removal of synthetic dyes from wastewaters: A review. Environment International. 2004;**30**(7):953-971

[17] Cripps C, Bumpus JA, Aust SD. Biodegradation of azo and heterocyclic

dyes by *Phanerochaete chrysosporium*. Applied and Environmental Microbiology. 1990;**56**(4):1114-1118

[18] Field JA, De Jong E, Costa GF, De Bont JAM. Biodegradation of polycyclic aromatic hydrocarbons by new isolates of white rot fungi. Applied and Environmental Microbiology. 1992;**58**(7):2219-2226

[19] Gupta S, Annepu SK, Summuna B, Gupta M, Nair SA. Role of mushroom fungi in decolourization of industrial dyes and degradation of agrochemicals. In: Biology of Macrofungi. Cham: Springer; 2018. pp. 177-190

[20] Freitag M, Morrell JJ. Decolorization of the polymeric dye Poly R-478 by wood-inhabiting fungi. Canadian Journal of Microbiology. 1992;**38**(8):811-822

[21] Moreno-Garrido I. Microalgae immobilization: Current techniques and uses. Bioresource Technology. 2008;**99**(10):3949-3964

[22] Yao J, Jia R, Zheng L, Wang B. Rapid decolorization of azo dyes by crude manganese peroxidase from Schizophyllum sp. F17 in solid-state fermentation. Biotechnology and Bioprocess Engineering. 2013;**18**(5): 868-877

[23] Lallawmsanga LVV, Passari AK, Muniraj IK, Uthandi S, Hashem A, et al. Elevated levels of laccase synthesis by *Pleurotus pulmonarius* BPSM10 and its potential as a dye decolorizing agent. Saudi Journal of Biological Sciences. 2019;**26**(3):464-468. DOI: 10.1016/j.sjbs.2018.10.006

[24] Chakraborty S, Basak B, Dutta S, Bhunia B, Dey A. Decolorization and biodegradation of congo red dye by a novel white rot fungus *Alternaria alternata* CMERI F6. Bioresource Technology. 2013;**147**:662-666

[25] Mahmoud MS. Decolorization of certain reactive dye from aqueous solution using Baker's Yeast (*Saccharomyces cerevisiae*) strain. HBRC Journal. 2016;**12**(1):88-98

[26] Sumandono T, Saragih H, Migirin, Watanabe T, Amirta R. Decolorization of remazol Brilliant Blue R by new isolated white rot fungus collected from tropical rain forest in East Kalimantan and its ligninolytic enzymes activity. Procedia Environmental Sciences. 2015;**28**:45-51

[27] Robinson T, McMullan G, Marchant R, Nigam P. Remediation of dyes in textile effluent: A critical review on current treatment technologies with a proposed alternative. Bioresource Technology. 2001;**77**(3):247-255

[28] Knapp JS, Newby PS, Reece LP. Decolorization of dyes by wood-rotting basidiomycete fungi. Enzyme and Microbial Technology. 1995;**17**(7): 664-668

[29] Tychanowicz GK, Zilly A, De Souza CGM, Peralta RM. Decolourisation of industrial dyes by solid-state cultures of Pleurotus pulmonarius. Process Biochemistry. 2004;**39**(7):855-859

[30] Kapoor A, Viraraghavan T. Removal of heavy metals from aqueous solutions using immobilized fungal biomass in continuous mode. Water Research. 1998;**32**(6):1968-1977

[31] Fu Y, Viraraghavan T. Removal of Congo Red from an aqueous solution by fungus *Aspergillus niger*. Advances in Environmental Research. 2002;**7**(1):239-247

[32] Arica MY, Bayramoğlu G. Biosorption of Reactive Red-120 dye from aqueous solution by native and modified fungus biomass preparations of *Lentinus sajor-caju*. Journal of Hazardous Materials. 2007;**149**(2):499-507

[33] Mou D-G, Lim KK, Shen HP. Microbial agents for decolorization

of dye wastewater. Biotechnology Advances. 1991;**9**(4):613-622. Available from: https://www.sciencedirect.com/science/article/pii/073497509190734D

[34] Demierege S, Toptas A, Mavioglu Ayan E, Yasa I, Yanik J. Removal of textile dyes from aqueous solutions by biosorption on mushroom stump wastes. Chemistry and Ecology. 2015;**31**(4):365-378. Available from: http://www.tandfonline.com/doi/full/10.1080/02757540.2014.976209

[35] Papinutti L, Forchiassin F. Adsorption and decolorization of dyes using solid residues from *Pleurotus ostreatus* mushroom production. Biotechnology and Bioprocess Engineering. 2010;**15**(6):1102-1109. Available from: http://link.springer.com/10.1007/s12257-010-0074-3

[36] Chen Z, Deng H, Chen C, Yang Y, Xu H. Biosorption of malachite green from aqueous solutions by *Pleurotus ostreatus* using Taguchi method. Journal of Environmental Health Science and Engineering. 2014;**12**(1):63

[37] Akar ST, Gorgulu A, Kaynak Z, Anilan B, Akar T. Biosorption of Reactive Blue 49 dye under batch and continuous mode using a mixed biosorbent of macro-fungus *Agaricus bisporus* and *Thuja orientalis* cones. Chemical Engineering Journal. 01 May 2009;**148**(1):26-34

[38] Pandey P, Singh RP, Singh KN, Manisankar P. Evaluation of the individuality of white rot macro fungus for the decolorization of synthetic dye. Environmental Science and Pollution Research. 2013;**20**(1):238-249. Available from: http://www.ncbi.nlm.nih.gov/pubmed/22467235

[39] Akar T, Anilan B, Kaynak Z, Gorgulu A, Akar ST. Batch and dynamic flow biosorption potential of *Agaricus bisporus/Thuja orientalis* biomass mixture for decolorization of RR45 dye. Industrial & Engineering Chemistry Research. 2008;**47**(23):9715-9723. Available from: https://pubs.acs.org/doi/10.1021/ie8007874

[40] Bayramoğlu G, Ozalp VC, Arıca MY. Removal of Disperse Red 60 dye from aqueous solution using free and composite fungal biomass of *Lentinus concinnus*. Water Science and Technology. 2017;**75**(2):366-377. Available from: https://iwaponline.com/wst/article/75/2/366-377/28696

[41] Grujić M, Dojnov B, Potočnik I, Duduk B, Vujčić Z. Spent mushroom compost as substrate for the production of industrially important hydrolytic enzymes by fungi Trichoderma spp. and *Aspergillus niger* in solid state fermentation. International Biodeterioration and Biodegradation. 2015;**104**:290-298

[42] Vyas BRM, Molitoris HP. Involvement of an extracellular H_2O_2-dependent ligninolytic activity of the white rot fungus *Pleurotus ostreatus* in the decolorization of Remazol brilliant blue R. Applied and Environmental Microbiology. 1995;**61**(11):3919-3927

[43] Kunjadia PD, Sanghvi GV, Kunjadia AP, Mukhopadhyay PN, Dave GS. Role of ligninolytic enzymes of white rot fungi (Pleurotus spp.) grown with azo dyes. SpringerPlus. 01 December 2016;**5**(1):1487

[44] dos Santos Bazanella GC, de Souza DF, Castoldi R, Oliveira RF, Bracht A, Peralta RM. Production of laccase and manganese peroxidase by *Pleurotus pulmonarius* in solid-state cultures and application in dye decolorization. Folia Microbiologia (Praha). 2013;**58**(6):641-647

[45] Cuamatzi-Flores J, Esquivel-Naranjo E, Nava-Galicia S, López-Munguía A, Arroyo-Becerra A, Villalobos-López MA, et al. Differential

regulation of Pleurotus ostreatus dye peroxidases gene expression in response to dyes and potential application of recombinant Pleos-DyP1 in decolorization. PLoS One. 2019;**14**(1): 209711

[46] Arunprasath T, Sudalai S, Meenatchi R, Jeyavishnu K, Arumugam A. Biodegradation of triphenylmethane dye malachite green by a newly isolated fungus strain. Biocatalysis and Agricultural Biotechnology. 2019;**17**(September):672-679. DOI: 10.1016/j.bcab.2019.01.030

[47] Copete LS, Chanagá X, Barriuso J, López-Lucendo MF, Martínez MJ, Camarero S. Identification and characterization of laccase-type multicopper oxidases involved in dye-decolorization by the fungus Leptosphaerulina sp. BMC Biotechnology. 2015;**15**(1):74

[48] Sivasakthivelan P. Decolorization of textile dyes and their effluents using white rot fungi. International Journal of ChemTech Research. 2013;**5**(3):1309-1312

[49] Prigione V, Tigini V, Pezzella C, Anastasi A, Sannia G, Varese GC. Decolourisation and detoxification of textile effluents by fungal biosorption. Water Research. 01 June 2008;**42**(12):2911-2920

[50] Gulzar T, Kiran S, Abrar S, Rahmat M, Haque A, Nosheen S, et al. Role of enzymatic system of screened *Pleurots ostreatus* IBL-02 in the bio-removal of synthetic dyes effluent. Journal of the Chemical Society of Pakistan. 2019;**41**(3):509-509. Available from: https://go.gale.com/ps/anonymous?id=GALE%7CA591700141&sid=googleScholar&v=2.1&it=r&linkaccess=abs&issn=02535106&p=AONE&sw=w

[51] Maria J, Silva MCS, Rodrigues M, Paes SA, Nunes MD, da Silva MDC, et al. Degradation of oxo-biodegradable plastic by degradation of oxo-biodegradable plastic by *Pleurotus ostreatus*. PLoS One. 2013;**8**(August):1-8

[52] Spadaro JT, Gold MH, Renganathan V. Degradation of azo dyes by the lignin-degrading fungus *Phanerochaete chrysosporium*. Applied and Environmental Microbiology. 1992;**58**(8):2397-2401

[53] Bumpus JA, Tien M, Wright D, Aust SD. Oxidation of persistent environmental pollutants by a white rot fungus. Science. 21 June 1985;**228**(4706):1434-1436

[54] Nilsson I, Möller A, Mattiasson B, Rubindamayugi MST, Welander U. Decolorization of synthetic and real textile wastewater by the use of white-rot fungi. Enzyme and Microbial Technology. 2006;**38**(1-2):94-100

[55] Paszczynski A, Crawford RL. Degradation of azo compounds by ligninase from *Phanerochaete chrysosporium*: Involvement of veratryl alcohol. Biochemical and Biophysical Research Communications. 1991;**178**(3):1056-1063

[56] Rodríguez CS. Dye removal by immobilised fungi. Biotechnology Advances. 01 May 2009;**27**(3):227-235

[57] Camacho-Morales RL, Sánchez JE. Biotechnological use of Fungi for the degradation of recalcitrant agro-pesticides. In: Mushroom Biotechnology. Academic Press; 01 January 2016. pp. 203-214

[58] Magan N, Fragoeiro S, Bastos C. Environmental factors and bioremediation of xenobiotics using white rot fungi. Mycobiology. 2010;**38**(4):238

[59] Subash SP, Chand P, Pavithra S, Balaji SJ, Pal S. Pesticide use in Indian agriculture: Trends, market structure and policy issues. 2017

[60] Kookana RS, Baskaran S, Naidu R. Pesticide fate and behaviour in Australian soils in relation to contamination and management of soil and water: A review. Australian Journal of Soil Research. 1998;**36**(5):715-764

[61] Nawaz K et al. Eco-friendly role of biodegradation against agricultural pesticides hazards. African Journal of Microbiology Research. 2011;**5**(3):177-183

[62] Hussain S, Siddique T, Arshad M, Saleem M. Bioremediation and phytoremediation of pesticides: Recent advances. Critical Reviews in Environmental Science and Technology. 09 October 2009;**39**(10):843-907

[63] Embrandiri A, Katheem Kiyasudeen S, Rupani PF, Ibrahim MH. Environmental xenobiotics and its effects on natural ecosystem. In: Plant Responses to Xenobiotics. Singapore: Springer; 2016. pp. 1-18

[64] Trejo-Hernandez MR, Lopez-Munguia A, Quintero RR. Residual compost of *Agaricus bisporus* as a source of crude laccase for enzymic oxidation of phenolic compounds. Process Biochemistry. 01 February 2001;**36**(7):635-639

[65] Agrawal N, Verma P, Shahi SK. Degradation of polycyclic aromatic hydrocarbons (phenanthrene and pyrene) by the ligninolytic fungi *Ganoderma lucidum* isolated from the hardwood stump. Bioresources and Bioprocessing. 2018;**5**(1):11

[66] da Luz JMR, Paes SA, Ribeiro KVG, Mendes IR, Kasuya MCM. Degradation of green polyethylene by *Pleurotus ostreatus*. PLoS One. 2015;**10**(6):e0126047

[67] Tsujiyama S, Muraoka T, Takada N. Biodegradation of 2,4-dichlorophenol by shiitake mushroom (*Lentinula edodes*) using vanillin as an activator. Biotechnology Letters. 01 July 2013;**35**(7):1079-1083

[68] Eskander SB, Abd El-Aziz SM, El-Sayaad H, Saleh HM. Cementation of bioproducts generated from biodegradation of radioactive cellulosic-based waste simulates by mushroom. ISRN Chemical Engineering. 29 November 2012;**2012**

[69] Yogita R, Simanta S, Aparna S, Kamlesh S. Biodegradation of malachite green by wild mushroom of Chhatisgrah. Journal of Experimental Sciences. 2011;**2**(10):69-72

[70] Olusola SA, Anslem EE. Bioremediation of a crude oil polluted soil with *Pleurotus pulmonarius* and *Glomus mosseae* using Amaranthus hybridus as a test plant. Journal of Bioremediation & Biodegradation. 2010;**1**(113):2155-6199

[71] Jang K-Y, Cho S-M, Seok S-J, Kong W-S, Kim G-H, Sung J-M. Screening of biodegradable function of indigenous ligno-degrading mushroom using dyes. Mycobiology. 01 March 2009;**37**(1):53-61

[72] Zebulun HO, Isikhuemhen OS, Inyang H. Decontamination of anthracene-polluted soil through white rot fungus-induced biodegradation. The Environmentalist. 01 March 2011;**31**(1):11-19

[73] Adedok OM, Ataga AE. Oil spills remediation using native mushroom—A viable option. Research Journal of Environmental Sciences. 01 January 2014;**8**(1):57

[74] Isikhuemhen OS, Anoliefo GO, Oghale OI. Bioremediation of crude oil polluted soil by the white rot fungus, *Pleurotus tuberregium* (Fr.) Sing. Environmental Science and Pollution Research. 01 March 2003;**10**(2):108-112

[75] Novotný C, Erbanová P, Cajthaml T, Rothschild N, Dosoretz C, Šašek V. *Irpex lacteus*, a white rot fungus applicable to water and soil bioremediation. Applied

Microbiology and Biotechnology. 2000;**54**(6):850-853

[76] Stella T, Covino S, Čvančarová M, Filipová A, Petruccioli M, D'Annibale A, et al. Bioremediation of long-term PCB-contaminated soil by white-rot fungi. Journal of Hazardous Materials. 15 February 2017;**324**:701-710

[77] Singh H. Mycoremediation: Fungal bioremediation. In: Mycoremediation: Fungal Bioremediation. John Wiley & Sons, Inc.; 17 November 2006

[78] Braun-Lüllemann A, Majcherczyk A, Hüttermann A. Degradation of styrene by white-rot fungi. Applied Microbiology and Biotechnology. 01 February 1997; **47**(2):150-155

[79] Patel H, Gupte A, Gupte S. Biodegradation of fluoranthene by basidiomycetes fungal isolate pleurotus ostreatus HP-1. Applied Biochemistry and Biotechnology. 01 June 2009;**157**(3):367

[80] Jackson MM, Hou L, Banerjee HN, Sridhar R, Dutta SK. Disappearance of 2,4-dinitrotoluene and 2-amino,4,6-dinitrotoluene by *Phanerochaete chrysosporium* under non-ligninolytic conditions. Bulletin of Environmental Contamination and Toxicology. 1999;**62**(4):390-396. Available from: http://www.ncbi.nlm.nih.gov/pubmed/10094719

[81] Bending GD, Friloux M, Walker A. Degradation of contrasting pesticides by white rot fungi and its relationship with ligninolytic potential. FEMS Microbiology Letters. 01 June 2002;**212**(1):59-63

[82] Alborés S, Pianzzola MJ, Soubes M, Cerdeiras MP. Biodegradation of agroindustrial wastes by Pleurotus spp for its use as ruminant feed. Electronic Journal of Biotechnology. June 2006;**9**(3)

[83] Belewu MA, Belewu KY. Cultivation of mushroom (*Volvariella volvacea*) on banana leaves. African Journal of. Biotechnology. 2005;**4**(12):1401-1403. Available from: http://www.academicjournals.org/AJB

[84] Lechner BE, Papinutti VL. Production of lignocellulosic enzymes during growth and fruiting of the edible fungus *Lentinus tigrinus* on wheat straw. Process Biochemistry. 01 March 2006;**41**(3):594-598

[85] Bilal M, Asgher M. Biodegradation of agrowastes by lignocellulolytic activity of an oyster mushroom, *Pleurotus sapidus*. Journal of the National Science Foundation of Sri Lanka. 2016;**44**(4):399-407

[86] Kuforiji OO, Fasidi IO. Enzyme activities of *Pleurotus tuber-regium* (Fries) Singer, cultivated on selected agricultural wastes. Bioresource Technology. 01 July 2008;**99**(10):4275-4278

[87] Rani P, Kalyani N, Prathiba K. Evaluation of lignocellulosic wastes for production of edible mushrooms. Applied Biochemistry and Biotechnology. 2008;**151**(2-3):151-159

[88] Kulshreshtha S, Mathur N, Bhatnagar P. Pros and cons of P. Florida cultivation for managing waste of handmade paper and cardboard industries. IIOAB Journal. 2011;**2**:45-48

[89] Akinyele JB, Fakoya S, Adetuyi CF. Anti-growth factors associated with *Pleurotus ostreatus* in a submerged liquid fermentation. Malaysian Journal of Microbiology. 2012;**8**:135-140

[90] Akinyele BJ, Olaniyi OO, Arotupin DJ. Bioconversion of selected agricultural wastes and associated enzymes by *Volvariella volvacea*: An edible mushroom. Research Journal of Microbiology. 2011;**6**(1):63-70

[91] Kulshreshtha S, Mathur N, Bhatnagar P. Mycoremediation of paper, pulp and cardboard industrial wastes and pollutants. In: Fungi as Bioremediator. Berlin, Heidelberg: Springer. 2013. pp. 77-116

[92] Kuforiji OO, Fasidi IO. Biodegradation of agro-industrial wastes by a edible mushroom Pleurotus tuber-regium (Fr.). Journal of Environmental Biology. 2009;**30**(3):355-358

[93] Brienzo M, Silva EM, Milagres AMF. Degradation of eucalypt waste components by *Lentinula edodes* strains detected by chemical and near-infrared spectroscopy methods. Applied Biochemistry and Biotechnology. 2007;**141**(1):37-49

[94] Shamim S. Biosorption of heavy metals. In: Biosorption. Rijeka: IntechOpen; 2018. Available from: http://www.intechopen.com/books/biosorption/biosorption-of-heavy-metals

[95] Thakur M. Mushrooms as a biological tool in mycoremediation of polluted soils. In: Emerging Issues in Ecology and Environmental Science. Cham: Springer; 2019. pp. 27-42

[96] Tay CC, Liew HH, Yin CY, Abdul-Talib S, Surif S, Suhaimi AA, et al. Biosorption of cadmium ions using *Pleurotus ostreatus*: Growth kinetics, isotherm study and biosorption mechanism. Korean Journal of Chemical Engineering. 2011;**28**(3):825-830

[97] Ibileye. Assessment of the Biosorption Potential of Heavy Metals by *Pleurotus tuber-regium* [Internet]. 2012. pp. 293-297. Available from: https://www.semanticscholar.org/paper/ASSESSMENT-OF-THE-BIOSORPTION-POTENTIAL-OF-HEAVY-BY-Ibileye/35357ef7a953b5d0b7de199ebc50f6128c2adedf

[98] Luo D, Xie YF, Tan ZL, Li XD. Removal of Cu^{2+} ions from aqueous solution by the abandoned mushroom compost of *Flammulina velutipes*. Journal of Environmental Biology. 01 April 2013;**34**(Suppl 2):359-365

[99] Lamrood Prasad Y, Ralengenker SD. Biosorption of Cu, Zn, Fe, Cd, Pb and Ni by non-treated biomass of some edible mushrooms. Asian Journal of Experimental Biological Sciences. 2014;**4**(2):190-195

[100] Sutherland CVC. Equilibrium modeling of Cu (II) biosorption onto untreated and treated forest macro-fungus *Fomes fasciatus*. International Journal of Plant, Animal and Environmental Sciences. 2015;**3**(1):193-203

[101] Nagy B, Măicăneanu A, Indolean C, Mânzatu C, Silaghi-Dumitrescu L, Majdik C. Comparative study of Cd(II) biosorption on cultivated *Agaricus bisporus* and wild *Lactarius piperatus* based biocomposites. Linear and nonlinear equilibrium modelling and kinetics. Journal of the Taiwan Institute of Chemical Engineers. 2014;**45**(3):921-929

[102] Fu Y, Viraraghavan T. Fungal decolorization of dye wastewaters: A review. Bioresource Technology. 01 September 2001;**79**(3):251-262

[103] Bellettini MB, Fiorda FA, Maieves HA, Teixeira GL, Ávila S, Hornung PS, et al. Factors affecting mushroom Pleurotus spp. Saudi Journal of Biological Sciences. 01 May 2019;**26**(4):633-646

[104] Velioglu Z, Ozturk Urek R. Optimization of cultural conditions for biosurfactant production by *Pleurotus djamor* in solid state fermentation. Journal of Bioscience and Bioengineering. 01 November 2015;**120**(5):526-531

[105] Chang ST, Miles PG. Mushrooms: Cultivation, nutritional value, medicinal effect, and

environmental impact. In: Mushrooms: Cultivation, Nutritional Value, Medicinal Effect, and Environmental Impact. 2nd ed. 2004

[106] Damodaran D, Shetty VB. Mushrooms in the remediation of heavy metals from soil. International Journal of Environmental Pollution Control and Management. 2011;**3**(1):89-101

[107] Boopathy R. Factors limiting bioremediation technologies. Bioresource Technology. 01 August 2000;**74**(1):63-67

[108] Singh DK. Biodegradation and bioremediation of pesticide in soil: Concept, method and recent developments. Indian Journal of Microbiology. 01 March 2008;**48**(1):35-40

[109] Árvay J, Tomáš J, Hauptvogl M, Kopernická M, Kováčik A, Bajčan D, et al. Contamination of wild-grown edible mushrooms by heavy metals in a former mercury-mining area. Journal of Environmental Science and Health, Part B. 2014;**49**(11):815-827. Available from: http://www.ncbi.nlm.nih.gov/pubmed/25190556

Chapter 7

Wild Medicinal Mushrooms: Potential Applications in Phytomedicine and Functional Foods

Clement Olusola Ogidi, Victor Olusegun Oyetayo and Bamidele Juliet Akinyele

Abstract

The accumulated secondary metabolites in medicinal mushrooms have been widely accepted as sources of safe and effective nutraceuticals, cosmeceuticals, and pharmaceuticals. Medicinal and edible mushrooms are foods appreciated for their exquisite flavor and medicinal properties. The nutritional values and biologically active compounds in mushrooms have immense potentials for producing new drugs of great health benefits to mankind. In recent times, medicinal mushrooms are being exploited for new and natural compounds that could modulate immune cell's response, and possess antimicrobial, antioxidants, and anticancer properties. In Nigeria, where there is vegetation that supports the luxuriant growth of varieties of naturally occurring macrofungi, some of the wild macrofungi have not been properly identified, adequately studied, and fully harnessed for their potentials as food and medicine. It is therefore pertinent to bring to limelight the nutraceutical potentials of some of these wild macrofungi that are currently underutilized.

Keywords: Nutraceuticals, medicinal mushrooms, mycochemicals, basidiomycetes

1. Introduction

Medicinal and edible mushrooms are mostly found in the higher basidiomycetes, and they usually have a saprophytic and aerobic growth habit, which allows them to grow on different lignocellulosic materials [1]. Fungi as a kingdom have very diverse group of living organisms found across all ecosystems [2]. Fungi are eukaryotes; they have microscopic organelles within their cells called nuclei which contain genetic materials in the form of threadlike chromosomes and enable hereditary characters to be passed on to subsequent generations [3]. The Basidiomycetes make up a colossal variety of fungi. Their taxonomic determination has been controversial and sometime challenging due to limited distinguishing characters and disagreement in features characteristics to be adopted for separating the different species [4]. The use of fruit body morphological characteristics such as appearance, color, dimension, spores and form of the fungus on pure culture, physiological factors, and environmental growth preferences can often mislead the identification of macrofungi without the use of microscopic examination coupled with molecular tools [5]. Therefore, the advancement and upsurge in the use of Deoxyribonucleic Acid (DNA) technology has proven to be a powerful tool for traditional taxonomic methods by solving the challenges of taxonomic chaos [6]. The rapid development with the use of versatile molecular techniques has provided easy approach, which is already being used to identify unknown basidiomycete isolates by comparing their DNA profiles with those fruit bodies that have been authenticated in GenBank. DNA techniques for the identification of fungi have been widely used in human and veterinary medicine; it is rapid and displays the accurate identity of pathogenic fungi in order to select appropriate treatment. They have also been applied to food quality control for the detection of contaminants [7]. The body or thallus of the basidiomycete fungus (the mycelium) is normally hidden within the substrate, and it is generally only the fruit body or basidiocarp that is visible at the surface. For this reason, the fruit body tends to show the greatest morphological variation. Conventional mycologists rely on a number of macroscopic and microscopic features of the fruit body to distinguish between macrofungi species [5].

2. Mushrooms

Mushrooms are foods that are commonly consumed since earliest history; ancient Greeks believed that mushrooms are a source of strength for warriors in battle; the Romans regard mushrooms as the "Food of the Gods" served them only on festive occasions. For centuries, the Chinese culture has treasured mushroom as a health food, an "elixir of life" [8]. Mushrooms are originally defined as macrofungi with a distinctive fruiting body, which is large enough to be seen with the naked eye and picked by hand [1]. They do not have the green pigment called chlorophyll that enables the plant to utilize energy from sunlight to change chemical into substances necessary for growth, a process commonly known as photosynthesis instead mushroom produces a wide range of extracellular enzymes [9]. This enables them to degrade complex organic matter into soluble substances, which can be absorbed for nutrition and stored as secondary metabolites [2]. The growth and fruiting of an individual mushroom species on particular substrate will depend upon their ability to produce enzymes that degrade the major component of the substrate such as cellulose, hemicelluloses, and ligin [10].

Macrofungi produce valuable enzymes and bioactive molecules with different therapeutic effects. Therefore, they are considered as flourishing organisms to develop different healthcare and biotechnological products [11]. Mushrooms have been a part of the human culture for thousands of years with considerable interest in civilization history because of their sensory characteristics and medicinal properties; they have been recognized for attractive culinary with low calories, carbohydrates, fat, and sodium with no amount of cholesterol [12, 13]. It has been estimated that there are about 140,000 species of mushrooms present on earth and only 5% are explored for uses, while 7000 were undiscovered species that could be of medicinal value to mankind [14]. With recent advances in medical and nutrition sciences, natural products from both edible and nonedible mushrooms have received extensive attention from individuals and health professionals due to the presence of biologically active compounds with denoted health benefits [15].

Owing to the increasing demand of natural bioactive compounds as an option to replace some synthetic drugs or additives in the pharmaceutical and food industries, the interest in fungi (medicinal mushrooms) has risen in recent years. The potential uses of the mushrooms have appeared as a nutraceutical, nutritional therapy, phytonutrients, phytotherapy, and pharmaceutical due to the accumulated number of secondary metabolites [16]. Several biologically active compounds such as polysaccharides (beta 1-3, 1-4, 1-6 glucans, hetero-beta glucans, proteo-glucans), krestin, lentinan, coriolan, schyzophillan, sesquiterpenes, quinones, hydrophobins, galectins, sterols, ergothionin, tri-teripenes, sterols, germanium, nucleotide, drosophilin, armillasin, amphalone, eloporoside, and volatile (skatole) were reported in medicinal mushrooms [17]. Mushrooms are the producers of extracellular proteolytic enzymes with fibrinolytic and thrombolytic activities [18]. Thus, the available information about bioactive molecules and enzymes in medicinal mushrooms suggests that they are promising candidate of choice microorganisms to develop health-enhancing biotechnological products. The presence of wide biomolecules in medicinal mushrooms has been attributed to different therapeutic effects such as antibacterial, antifungal, cytotoxic, antiinflammatory, insecticidal, nematocidal, and antioxidant [19].

2.1 Lifecycle of higher fungi (macrofungi)

The lifecycle of basidiomycetes includes special stages such as the alternation of generations [3]. Spores from basidium are generally produced for sexual reproduction, rather than asexual reproduction [20]. The club-shaped basidium carries spores called basidiospores. In the basidium, nuclei of two different mating strains (− and +) fuse (karyogamy), giving rise to a diploid zygote that then undergoes meiosis as shown in **Figure 1**. The haploid nuclei migrate into basidiospores, which germinate and generate monokaryotic hyphae. The mycelium that results is called a primary mycelium. Mycelia of different mating strains can combine and produce a secondary mycelium that contains haploid nuclei of two different mating strains. This is the dikaryotic stage of the basidiomycetes lifecycle, which also referred to as dominant stage. Eventually, the secondary mycelium generates a basidiocarp,

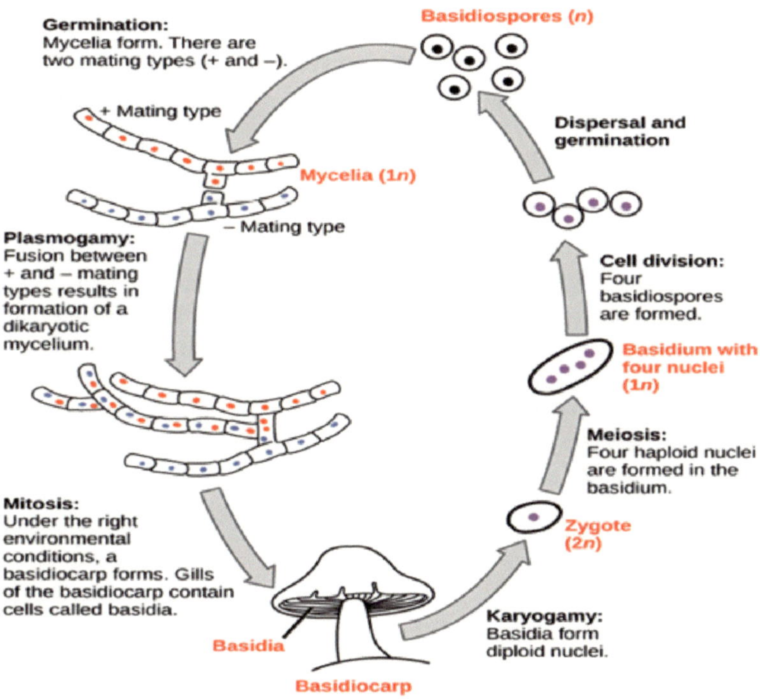

Figure 1.
Reproductive stages of Basidiomycetes: macrofungi [5].

a fruiting body that protrudes either above the soil (epigeous macrofungi) as the basidiocarp bears the developing basidia on the gills under its cap at depths of 10–20 cm or below the soil surface as hypogeous macrofungi or truffles. In the phylum Basidiomycota, sexual reproduction is often dictated by two independent sets of mating-type specific genes, which control the stages of the sexual cycle. The genes encode premating lipopeptide pheromones and their cognate receptors mediate the recognition of mating partners, cell fusion, and homeodomain transcription factors, which form heterodimers to regulate postmating behavior. Sexual reproduction in many fungal species has a central role in pathogenic development, promoting genetic variation, adaptation to fluctuating environments, and a long-term survival [21].

3. Examples of some wild and medicinal mushrooms

3.1 *Ganoderma* species

It is a polypore mushroom, which grows on wood. *Ganoderma* can be differentiated from other polypores because they have a double-walled basidiospore. The name *Ganoderma* is derived from the Greek *ganos* "brightness-sheen" or "shining" and *derma* "skin" [22]. *Ganoderma* is characterized by basidiocarps that are large, perennial, and woody brackets, also called "conks." They are lignicolous, leathery either with or without a stem. The fruit bodies typically grow in a fanlike or hooflike form on the trunks of living or dead trees. They have double-walled, truncate spores with yellow to brown ornamented inner layers. The genus was named by Karsten in 1881. Members of the family Ganodermataceae were traditionally considered difficult to classify because of the lack of reliable morphological characteristics, the genus was divided into two sections: *Ganoderma* with a shiny cap surface as *G. lucidum* and Elfvingia with a dull cap surface as *G. aapplanatum* [23]. Phylogenetic analysis using DNA sequence information derived from mitochondrial Small Subunit (SSU) rDNA has helped to clarify our understanding of the relationships among *Ganoderma* species. The genus may now be divided into some monophyletic group, namely *G. colossus*, *G. applanatum*, *G. tsugae*, Asian *G. lucidum* group, *G. meredithiae*, and *G. resinaceum* [24].

3.2 *Rigidoporus* species

The fungi form many white, somewhat flattened mycelia strand of 1–2 mm thick that grow on and adhere strongly to the surface of the root bark. *Rigidoporus microporus* is a broad fruit body (20 cm wide), leathery, faintly velvety, broadly attached shelf, and often imbricate with the substrate. Their color ranged from orange to red or brown and later faded [25]. These rhizomorphs grow rapidly and may extend several meters through the soil in the absence of any woody substrate. Thus, healthy rubber trees can be infected by free rhizomorphs growing from stumps or infected woody debris buried in the ground as well as by roots contacting those of a diseased neighboring tree [26].

3.3 *Tremella* species

Tremella spp. belong to the family Tremellaceae. *Tremella* spp. are parasites of other fungi and most produce anamorphic yeast states when Basidiocarps (fruit bodies) are produced; they are gelatinous and colloquially classed among the "jelly fungi." Over 100 species of *Tremella* are currently recognized worldwide. Two species namely: *T. fuciformis* and *T. aurantialba* are commercially cultivated for food [27]. The name comes from the Latin *tremere* means "to tremble." Linnaeus placed *Tremella* in the algae including seaweeds, cyanobacteria, and myxomycetes as well as fungi, but Persoon revised *Tremella* in 1794 and 1801. He repositioned and considered *Tremella* as a genus (*Tremella* Pers.) from the originally created by Linnaeus (*Tremella* L.). *Tremella* Pers. has now been conserved under the International Code of Botanical Nomenclature with *Tremella mesenterica* as a species [28]. *Tremella* species produce hyphae that are typically (but not always) clamped and have haustorial cells, which penetrate the hyphae of the host. The basidia are "tremelloid," occur in globose to ellipsoid with vertically or diagonally septate. Conidiophores are often present and similar to yeast cells [28]. *Tremella mesenterica* occurs widely in broadleaf and mixed forests. It is widely distributed in temperate and tropical regions, which include Africa, Asia, Australia, Europe, and North and South America. Although considered bland and flavorless, the fungus is edible. *Tremella mesenterica* produce bioactive compounds that are attracting research interest because of their various biological activities [29].

3.4 *Agaricus* species

It is an important genus of mushroom containing both edible and poisonous species with over 300 members worldwide. The genus includes the common (button) mushroom (*Agaricus bisporus*) and field mushroom (*Agaricus campestris*). Members of *Agaricus* are characterized by having a fleshy cap (pileus) from the underside gills that produced the naked spores [30]. Members of *Agaricus* also have a stem (stipe), which elevates the pileus above the substrate and a partial veil and protects the developing gills and later forms a ring on the stalk [31]. *Agaricus* spp. are known as the most common mushroom with different names: button mushroom, white mushroom, table mushroom, champignon mushroom, crimini mushroom, Swiss brown mushrooms, Roman brown mushrooms, and Italian mushroom.

3.5 *Grifola frondosa*

It is a polypore mushroom that grows in clusters at the base of trees, particularly oaks. The fruiting body of *G. frondosa* occurs as large as 60 cm; it has a cluster consisting of multiple grayish-brown caps that are often curled or spoon-shaped with wavy margins of 2–7 cm broad. The undersurface of each cap bears approximately 1–3 pores per millimeter with the tubes rarely deeper than 3 mm. The milky-white stipe (stalk) has a branchy structure and becomes tough as the mushroom matures. *G. frondosa* is a perennial fungus that often grows in the same place for a number of years in succession. It is prized in traditional Chinese and Japanese herbology as a medicinal mushroom due to the ability to balance out altered body systems into a normal level. Most Japanese find it tasty and the texture is enormously appealing, though the mushroom has been alleged to cause allergic reactions in rare cases and becomes inedible such as all polypores when they are older because it is too tough to eat [33].

3.6 *Lentinus* species

It is a genus of fungi in the family Polyporaceae and widely spread in subtropical regions [34]. *Lentinus* spp. possess extracellular enzymes and thus act as wood-decaying basidiomycetes, gregarious on fallen wood of a wide variety of deciduous trees such as shii, oak, chestnut, beech, maple, sweetgum, cotton, alder, hornbeam, ironwood, chinquapin, and mulberry in a warm or moist climate [35]. The geographic distribution of *L. edodes* (Shiitake) in nature is widely extended through the various continents such as Asia, Europe, Australia, Africa, and America, and often time it is utilized as a medicinal food [34]. The genus name, *Lentinus*, is derived from the Latin *lent*, meaning "pliable," and *inus*, meaning "resembling." Pegler [36] correlated morphological differences with geographic distribution to recognize three species of shiitake: *Lentinus lateritia* in Southeast Asia and Australasia and *Lentinus novaezelandieae* in New Zealand. Other species of *Lentinus* include: *L. crinitus* and *L. tigrinus* [35].

3.7 *Calocybe indica*

Calocybe indica, commonly known as the milky-white mushroom, is a species of edible mushroom native to India. The sturdy all-white mushrooms appear in summer after rainfall in fields (grassland), on road verges, and generally on substrate rich in organic material. It is being grown commercially in several Indian states and other tropical countries and traditionally eaten in West Bengal for medicinal purposes [37]. The robust mushroom is all-white in color and has a firm consistency. Its cap is 10–14 cms (4–5 $^{1}/_{2}$ in) across, convex initially before flattening out with age. The cuticle (skin) can be easily peeled off the cap. The crowded gills are white, and the cylindrical stem is 10 cms (4 in) high with no ring nor volva. It has a subbulbous base, being 1.8 cms ($^{3}/_{4}$ in) wide at the apex (top), 3.5 cms (1 $^{1}/_{2}$ in) in the middle, and 2.4 cms (1 in) wide at the base. The mushroom does not change color on cutting or bruising, though old dried specimens have a buff color. The flesh has a mild flavor that has been described as oily, and a faint smell reminiscent of radishes. The spore print is white, and the oval spores measure 5.9–6.8 μm long by 4.2–5.1 μm wide [37]. The mushrooms appear between May and August after spells of rainfall. The fungus is saprophytic, though it has been reported to form ectomycorrhizal relationships with the roots of the coconut tree (*Cocos nucifera*), palmyra palm (*Borassus flabellifer*), tamarind (*Tamarindus indicus*), and yellow poinciana (*Peltophorum pterocarpum*) [37].

3.8 *Pleurotus ostreatus*

Pleurotus ostreatus, the oyster mushroom, is a common edible mushroom. It was first cultivated in Germany as a subsistence measure during World War [38] and is now grown commercially around the world for food. It is related to the similarly cultivated king oyster mushroom. Oyster mushrooms can also be used industrially for mycoremediation purposes, it attacks and kills nematodes and bacteria with impunity. The oyster mushroom is one of the more commonly sought wild mushrooms, though it can also be cultivated on straw and other media. It has the bittersweet aroma of benzaldehyde [38]. *Pleurotus ostreatus* is easily recognized by the way it grows on wood in shelflike clusters; its relatively large size; its whitish gills that run down a stubby, nearly absent stem; and its whitish to lilac spore print. It appears between October and early April across North America and features a brown cap. A number of very similar species are closely related, including *P. pulmonarius* (which is often paler and appears between late April and September) and *P. populinus* (which is found in the wood of quaking aspen). The mushroom has a broad, fan, or oyster-shaped cap spanning of 5–25 cms; natural specimens range from white to gray or tan to dark-brown; the margin is enrolled when young, and is smooth and often somewhat lobed or wavy. The flesh is white, firm, and varies in thickness due to stipe arrangement. The gills of the mushroom are white to cream and descend on the stalk if present. If so, the stipe is off-center with a lateral attachment to wood. The spore print of the mushroom is white to lilac-gray and best viewed on dark background. The mushroom's stipe is often absent. When present, it is short and thick [39]. It is mainly saprophytic but can be a facultative parasite on a stressed host. Sporophytes can be found growing naturally on both living and dead trees of a wide array of broadleaf hardwoods and conifers. Many different subspecies, varieties, and strains can be found within this species, but there are two major ecotypes: brown forms from North America and blue/brown forms from Europe [40].

3.9 *Lenzites* species

Lenzites spp. are wood-decaying fungi in the class Agaricomycetes, order Polyporale, family Polyporaceae, and genus *Lenzites*. *Lenzites* spp. were circumscribed by Elias Magnus Fries in 1835 and reportedly found in parts of Europe, Asia, and Africa [41]. The species is a white-rot pathogen living on woods; it has corky fruiting bodies in the shape of semicircular plates formed on the trunks of several types of deciduous trees. The fruiting body has a lamellar fruit layer (gills) producing spores. The upper surface of the cap may be in various shades of brown and sometimes zonate. The pore surface is white to tan at initial stage but as the fruit body matures, some of the pore walls break down, forming slits with blunt partitions. This results in the characteristic of a mazelike (daedaloid or labyrinthinine/labyrinthiform) appearance. The tube walls are 10–30 mm long with thick walls. The basidiospores are within 6–8 μm, smooth and elliptical in shape [42]. *Lenzites* spp. are widely available and index fungorum has reported 26 species [43].

The three synonymous wood-rotting fungi, namely: *Lenzites* spp., *Daedalea* spp., and *Trametes* spp., have been screened as cellulose-degraders from 20 different genera of both brown and white-rotters of Polyporaceae on the basis of their potential to degrade carboxymethylcellulose. The utilization of different carbon sources in the growth medium was studied with these fungi for the identification of enzymes involved in saccharification. Carboxymethyl cellulose and beta-glucosidase were identified as the two major enzymes involved in this process. Extracellular carboxymethyl cellulose from *L. saepiaria* has been purified to homogeneity and the enzyme partially characterized [44]. *Lenzites* spp. have been investigated for bioremediation application, production of laccase—a lignin-degrading enzyme, which has been isolated and purified for the production of various dyes, pigments, and bio pulping to eliminate the pollution hazards associated with the use of chlorine pulping process [45]. They have been used as a natural comb for brushing down hair of horses, and fruit bodies were used for anesthetizing bees [46]. *Lenzites* spp. are also known to have some medicinal properties, including antioxidant, antimicrobial, antitumor, and immunosuppressive activities, but only few species such *as L. betulina* and *L. warnieri* have been examined and documented [47].

4. Health benefits of edible and medicinal mushrooms

4.1 Nutritional benefits

Mushrooms contain the amino acids, vitamins, macro, microelements, and a substantial amount of dietary fibers. Higher Basidiomycetes have much insoluble dietary fiber bound with chitin, hemicellulose, mannans, glucans, glycogen, and trehalose in their cell wall. Cheung [48] has reported the health benefits of dietary fiber, which include the following: relieves of constipation, prevention of colon disease and hemorrhoids as well maximize the viscosity of the food matrix, slow-down of digestion, lower blood glucose, and strengthens immune system with antitumor activity. Mushrooms are excellent sources of dietary fiber, which can be used for the enrichment of biopharmaceutical products [49]. Mushrooms are known to possess complexes of polysaccharides and protein, which enhance innate and cell-mediated immune responses and exhibit antitumor activities in animals and humans [50]. Edible and medicinal mushrooms contain considerable amount of essential and nonessential amino acids. Essential fatty acid (linoleic acid), a precursor of 1-octen-3-ol, has been the principal active compound that contributed to the aroma and flavor of mushrooms. The bioavailability of mineral in medicinal mushrooms, except sodium in low concentrations, has made edible mushrooms choice of food that regulate blood pressure, maintain cellular function, and promote the availability of metalloenzymes, biochemical processes, and metabolic growth [51, 52].

The nutrient contents of various edible mushrooms play a vital role in maintaining the normal function of human body [53]. The utilization of macrofungi as a nutritional source provides opportunity to fulfill the protein-energy demand and thus balance the problem of nutritional deficiency [12]. Hence, it has been well proven and documented in the world literature that mushrooms provide definite nutrition and health benefits for humans. Nowadays, people eat mushrooms as functional foods, food-flavoring material in soups or sauces due to their unique and subtle flavor with devoid of undesirable side effects. The reason behind the consumption of mushrooms since ancient times is due to their nutritional benefits, organoleptic values, and pharmacological applications [54]. Badalyan [55] reported a significant reduction of blood cholesterol levels when lovastatin from submerged mycelia of *Pleurotus ostreatus* and *P. eryngii* var. *ferulae* was used as a dietary supplement. It needs to be noted that edible and some medicinal macrofungi are used as food, medicine, and formulated feeds for animals [56, 57].

4.2 Immunomodulatory activity

The combination of vitamins A, B, C complex, fiber, minerals, and other bioactive compounds in mushroom is a basic healing requirement to improve the human immune system against bacteria, fungi, and virus infections. *Ganoderma lucidum* contains a high concentration of organic germanium, polysaccharides, and triterpenes; these active components have been proven to strength, regulate immune system, and eliminate allergic reactions such as asthma, rheumatoid, arthritis, and lupus [58]. Findings of Zhu et al. [59] revealed that the bioactive compounds in edible and medicinal mushroom improve blood circulation, increase the activities of immune cells such as macrophages, natural killer cells (NK), and T-cells, and therefore reduce the tumor formation by 86%. *Lentinus edodes* contains lentinan that stimulates the production of immune system such as interleukin and tumor necrosis factor (TNF) which help to prevent the spread of cancer [60].

G. lucidum stimulated the production of interleukin-II due to the presence of ganoderic acid, which is active against liver cancer [61]. Medicinal mushrooms help in fighting infection as they stimulate the maturation of macrophage cells that engulf and neutralize bacteria particularly secondary infection [62]. Most importantly, mushrooms contain a large selection of biologically active polysaccharides, which are known to function as biological response modifiers (BRM). Biological response modifiers are substances that stimulate the body's response to infections and diseases. They contain repetitive structural features that are the polymer of monosaccharides residues joined to each other by glycosidic linkage [63, 64]. This offers a high capacity for carrying biological information because of their structural variability, ability to interconnect at several points to create a wide array of linear and branched molecules that will carry different biological information [65].

4.3 Anticancer properties

Cancer is medically known as malignant neoplasm—a disease involving unregulated cell growth [66]. Cancer is a devastating disease that may spread to more distant parts of the body through the lymphatic system or bloodstream. It afflicts many people around the world because it is the second leading cause of death after heart disease [67]. Several studies from Asian countries show that edible and medicinal mushrooms played an important role in the prevention and treatment of cancer [68]. In Eastern Europe, fruiting bodies of *Inonotus obliquus* have been used as a medicine for the treatment of cancer due to the presence of triterpenes and ergosterol peroxide [17]. The antitumor effect of several extracts and isolated compounds from mushrooms have been carried out on tumor cells and in animal assay [30]. The clinical evidence for anticancer activity of medicinal mushroom comes from the extracted polysaccharides, lentinan, PSK (Krestin), or schizophyllan [50].

Mushrooms prevent breast and prostate cancer due to the presence of beta-glucans and conjugated linoleic acid [69]. Anticarcinogenic effects of linoleic acid had been attributed to the ability to suppress estrogen [70]. *Agaricus bisporus, Lentinus edodes*, and *Grifola frondosa* possess bioactive substances that inhibit the activity of aromatase—an enzyme involved in estrogen production, which is a prime reason for breast cancer in the woman after menopause [71]. Other wild mushrooms such as *Pleurotus* spp., *Agaricus blazei*, *Ganoderma lucidum*, *Clitocybe nebularis, Trametes* spp., *Piptoporus betulinus*, *Inocybe umbrinella*, *Coprinus comatus*, *Fomes fomentarius*, *Lactarius flavidulus*, *Albatrellus confluens, Cordyceps sinensis, Schizophyllum commune*, and *Inonotus obliquus* have **Figure 2** been credited with anticancer activity due to some bioactive compounds [72].

4.4 Antimicrobial properties

The development of new synthetic antimicrobial compounds has led to a drastic increase in bacterial resistance and the subsequent evolution of multidrug-resistance among microorganisms [73]. In the quest for effective and sustainable antimicrobial substances against pathogenic microorganisms, a new group of microorganisms has been increasingly studied, among which mushrooms have emerged as a viable source of new antimicrobials [74]. Mushrooms need antibacterial and antifungal compounds as a defensive tool to survive in their natural environment. It is therefore not surprising that antimicrobial compounds could be isolated from many mushrooms for human benefits [50]. Sesquiterpenoid and hydroquinones produced by the *Ganoderma pfeiffer* inhibited the growth of Methicillin-resistant *Staphylococcus aureus* [75]. The extracts obtained from *L. quercina* inhibited the growth of *S. epidermidis*, *S. saprohyticus*, and *S. aureus* isolated from stool, urine and wound infections [76]. Applanoxidic acid isolated from *G. annulare* (Fr) shows antifungal activity against *Trichophyton mentagrophytes*, while the ethanolic extract of *L. edodes* was reported to possess antiprotozoal activity against *Paramecium caudatum* [77]. Ganoderic acid, ganodermadiol, ganodermanotriol, lucidadiol, triterpenes, and applaanoxidic acid isolated from *Ganoderma* species have been reported to possess in vitro antiviral activity against human immunodeficiency virus type I (HIV-1) and influenza virus type A [78]. Water-soluble lignin isolated from *Inonstus obliqueis* inhibited HIV protease; the

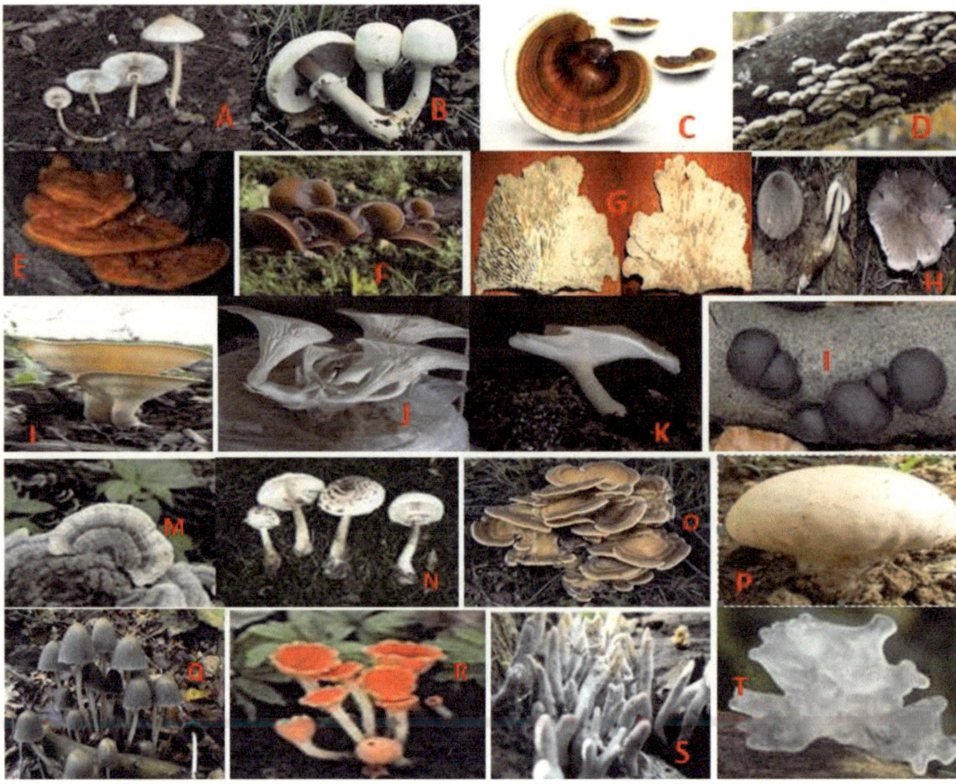

Figure 2.
Examples of some medicinal mushrooms in Nigeria [32]. A: Macrolepiota sp. B: Agaricus arvensis. C: Ganoderma lucidum. D: Schizophyllum commune. E: Pycnoporus cinnabarinus. F: Auricularia auricula. G: Lenzites quercina. H: Termitomyces. I: Pleurotus tuber-regium. J: Pleurotus ostreatus. K: Lentinus squarrosulus. L: Daldinia concentrica. M: Trametes versicolor. N: Chloropyllum sp. O: Meripilus giganteus. P: Lycoperdon spadiceum. Q: Coprinus lagopides. R: Microstoma sp. S: Xylaria hypoxylon. T: Tremella fuciformis.

protein-bound polysaccharides from *Trametes versicolor* (L. fr) have antiviral effect against HIV and cytomegalovirus. Antiviral agents from different mushroom species such as *Piptoporus betulinus*, *Fomitopsis officinalis*, and *Coprinellus micaceus* have been tested against different viruses, namely: Papilloma, infleuza (H5N1), Hepatitis B, C, D, and E [17]. El-Fakharany et al. [79] reported that a laccase has been purified from *P. ostreatus* mushroom, which is capable to inhibit the hepatitis C virus entry into peripheral blood cells and hepatoma HepG2 cells and its replication, whereas the isolation of a novel ubiquitinlike protein from *P. ostreatus* mushrooms manifests an inhibitory activity toward HIV-1 reverse transcriptase [80].

Studies carried out by Karacsonyi and Kuniak [81] revealed that beta-D Glucan (pleuran) isolated from fruiting bodies of *P. ostreatus* promoted the survival of mice susceptible to bacterial infections. Phenolic and tannin constituents of *P. ostreatus* may also elicit antibacterial activity through various mechanisms of action characterized by cell membrane lysis, inhibition of protein synthesis, proteolytic enzymes, and microbial adhesins [82]. The oil of the macrofungus extracted with petroleum ether and acetone was observed to inhibit the Gram-positive and Gram-negative bacterial tested in vitro to suggest that *P. ostreatus* has a broad-spectrum antibacterial activity [82], whereas organic extracts (methanol and chloroform) of *P. ostreatus* have been manifested as effective against Gram-positive bacteria which showed to be a potential source of antibacterial agents [83]. Comparative studies were carried out on the antibacterial activity of *P. ostreatus* and biosynthesized silver nanoparticles using *P. ostreatus* against Gram-positive bacteria using standard zones of inhibition, in which synthesized silver nanoparticles using *P. ostreatus* showed maximum zone of inhibition [84].

4.5 Antioxidant properties

The interplay between free radicals, antioxidants, and cofactors is important in maintaining stable health and age-related diseases [85]. Free radicals induce oxidative stress, which is balanced by the body's endogenous antioxidant system with input from cofactors and by the ingestion of exogenous antioxidants [86]. When the generation of free radicals exceeds the protective effect of antioxidants and some cofactors, it can cause oxidative damage, which can result in aging and other diseases such as cardiovascular, cancer, and neurodegenerative disorders [87]. The progressive severe and chronic disorders caused by free radicals have led to alternative sources of antioxidants compounds from wild mushrooms, which could be a remedy to dietetic aliments [88]. Hence, there is an emerging interest in the use of naturally occurring antioxidants for the preservation of foods, in other to manage a number of pathophysiological conditions.

Epidemiological studies have consistently shown that a high dietary intake of mushrooms is strongly associated with the reduced risk of developing chronic diseases such as cancer and cardiovascular disease [89]. This suggests that changes in dietary intake and consumption of natural foods provide desirable health benefits beyond basic nutrition to reduce the risk of chronic diseases. Medicinal mushrooms such as the species of *Termitomycetes*, *Pleurotus*, *Lentinus*, and *Lenzites* have shown potent scavenging properties against free radicals [90]. Generally, mushrooms contain ergothioneine, a naturally occurring and powerful antioxidant that protects the body's cells from generated free radicals as well as boost up immunity [91, 92]. The antioxidant activity of macrofungi had been attributed to the presence of useful metabolites in medicinal mushrooms. Therefore, the bioactive compounds in wild medicinal mushrooms make them a good source of antioxidant compounds to prevent degenerative diseases such as cardiovascular illnesses, neurodegenerative disorders, rheumatoid arthritis, and cancer that had been attributed to generated free radicals in the body.

Mushroom is an ideal low energy diet for diabetics; it has no fats, no cholesterol, very low carbohydrates, moderate protein, vitamins, minerals, dietary fibers, and a lot of water [48]. Moreover, mushrooms contain natural insulin and enzyme that break down sugar or starch [93]. *Diabetes mellitus* is a metabolic disorder affecting a large number of people [94]. Therefore, more effective and safer treatment for diabetes patients needs to be investigated in order to overcome the peripheral of insulin resistance. A polysaccharide fraction of *Grifola frondosa* (SX fraction) has been reported to exhibit hypoglycemic action in patients with type 2 diabetes [60]. Coriolan, glucans, ganoderan A and B from *Ganoderma lucidum*, and glucuronoxylomannan from the fruit bodies of *Tremella mesenterica* exhibited hypoglycemic effects in several tests and ameliorated the symptoms of diabetes (**Figure 3**) [95].

4.6 Antidiabetes properties

Many medicinal mushrooms have been found to be suitable for diabetic and heart patients due to low starch and low cholesterol content. Several mushroom species have been reported to be effective for both the control of blood glucose levels and the modification of the course of diabetic complications. This is because they are known to contain bioactive components that help with the proper functioning of metabolic organs such as the liver, pancreas, and other endocrinal glands,

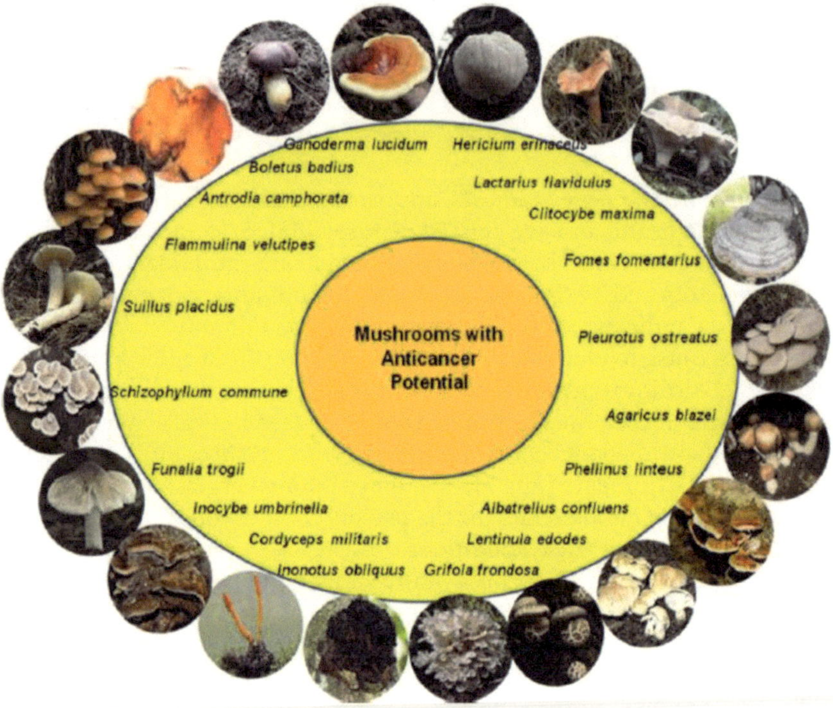

Figure 3.
Some medicinal mushrooms with nutraceutical potentials [72].

thereby promoting the formation of insulin and related hormones that ensure healthy metabolic functioning [50]. Mushrooms contain polysaccharides such as beta-glucans which can restore the function of pancreatic tissues eventually triggering increased insulin output by beta-cells, thus leading to decrease blood glucose levels. Beta-glucans have been shown to improve the sensitivity of peripheral tissues to insulin [96].

5. Underutilization of medicinal mushrooms in Nigeria

Most of the wild macrofungi found in Nigeria **Figure 2** are similar to mushrooms reported to possess anticancer properties [72]. One of the wild mushrooms from Nigeria—*Lenzites quercina* displayed anticancer activity against Hela and RD cell lines (**Figures 4** and **5**) in our latest findings [97, 98]. In recent studies, researchers had focused on the maximum utilization of natural bioactive compounds from edible and medicinal mushrooms **Figure 6**. Few species of medicinal mushrooms have been examined for anticancer activities in Nigeria. This may due to the lack of information on the identity and anticancer activities of available wild species of mushrooms.

Despite the millennial existence and empirical documentation of mushrooms, the ethnological knowledge of macrofungi, historical uses of mushrooms as food, medicine, source of income, and sociological impacts are apparently dawdling the ethnomycology research drive in Nigeria [99]. The poor identification and documentation of medicinal and edible mushrooms have created some degrees of inconsistencies in their usages relatively to the medicinal practice, food, and mythological beliefs [100]. The random utilization of mushrooms, the limited scope of taxonomic

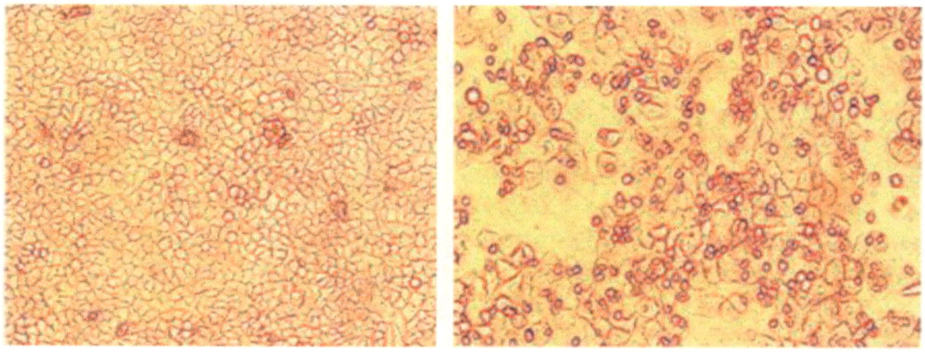

Figure 4.
Anticancer activity of Lenzites quercina extract against HeLa (a) cell line (HeLa) without extract and (b) cell line (HeLa) with extract at 100 μg.

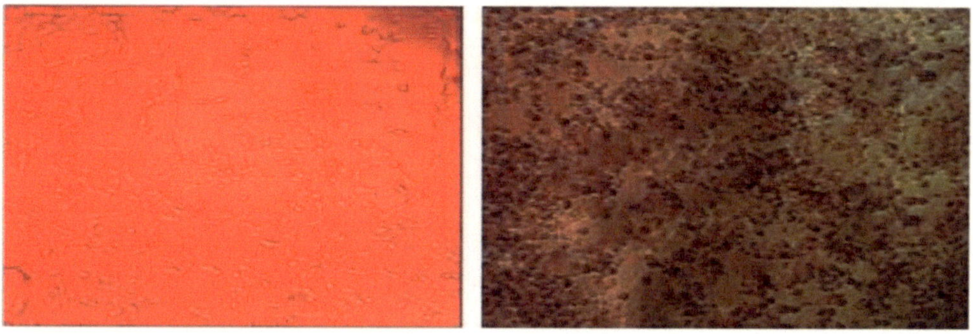

Figure 5.
Anticancer activity of Lenzites quercina extract against RD (a) cell line (RD) without extract and (b) cell line (RD) with extract at 100 μg.

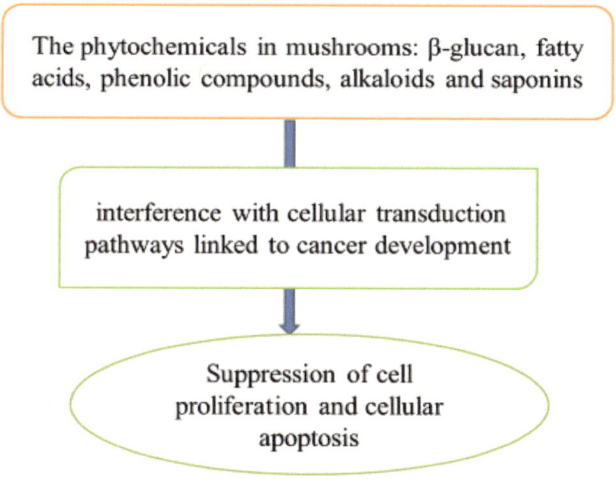

Figure 6.
Effect of bioactive compounds in medicinal mushroom on cancer cell lines.

consistencies of the existing mushroom, anthropogenic, ethnographic, ethnoecological, and religion have hindered the correct estimate of macrofungi for proper utilization and exploration in Nigeria and Africa.

6. Conclusion

The relevance of medicinal mushrooms in modern-day pharmaceuticals and nutraceuticals is an innovative conception in medical fields and food industries. The positive transformation of mushrooms into edible foods or products requires government support by sponsoring programs to assist agricultural development in mushroom isolation, identification, cultivation, and utilization. This could be a means to diversifying into food production to solve the food insecurity and as well deconcentrate the economic reliance on crude oil.

Author details

Clement Olusola Ogidi[1]*, Victor Olusegun Oyetayo[2] and Bamidele Juliet Akinyele[2]

1 Biotechnology Unit, Department of Biological Sciences, Kings University, Odeomu, Nigeria

2 Department of Microbiology, The Federal University of Technology, Akure, Nigeria

*Address all correspondence to: clementogidi@yahoo.com

References

[1] Chang ST, Miles PG. Mushroom biology–A new discipline. The Mycologist. 1992;**6**:64-65

[2] Prescott LM, Flarley JP, Klevin OA. Microbiology. 6th ed. New York: McGraw-Hill Education; 2010

[3] Alexopoulos CJ, Mims CW, Blackwell MM. Introductory Mycology. 4th ed. New York: John Wiley; 1996

[4] Guarro J, Gene J, Stchigel AM. Developments in fungal taxonomy. Clinical Microbiology Reviews. 1999; **12**(3):454-500

[5] Hood IA. The mycology of the Basidiomycetes. In: Heart Rot and Root Rot in Tropical *Acacia* Plantations. Proceedings of a Workshop Held in Yogyakarta, Indonesia. Vol. 124. Canberra: Australian Center for International Agricultural Research (ACIAR); 2006. pp. 34-59

[6] Min XJ, Hickey DA. Assessing the effect of varying sequence length on DNA barcoding of Fungi. Molecular Ecology Notes. 2007;**7**: 365-373

[7] Bauer R, Begerow D, Sampaio JP, Weib M, Oberwinkler F. The simple-septate Basidiomycetes: A synopsis. Mycological Progress. 2006;**5**:41-66

[8] Chang ST, Miles PG. Mushrooms-Cultivation, Nutritional Value, Medicinal Effect and Environmental Impact. 2nd ed. Boca Raton, London: CRC Press; 2004. pp. 2-4

[9] Leo VV, Passari AK, Joshi JB, Mishra VK, Uthandi S, Gupta VK, et al. A novel triculture system (CC_3) for simultaneous enzyme production and hydrolysis of common grasses through submerged fermentation. Frontiers in Microbiology. 2016;**7**:447

[10] Lallawmsanga LVV, Passari AK, Muniraj IK, Uthandi S, Hashem A, Abd-Allah EF, et al. Elevated levels of laccase synthesis by *Pleurotus pulmonarius* BPSM10 and its potential as a dye decolorizing agent. Saudi Journal of Biological Sciences. 2018;**26**(3): 464-468

[11] Singh BP, Chhakchhuak L, Passari AK, editors. Biology of Macrofungi. Switzerland: Springer International Publisher; 2018. DOI: 10.1007/978-3-030-02622-6

[12] Heleno SA, Barros L, Anabela M, Patricia M, Virginia FR, Jasmina G, et al. Nutritional value, bioactive compounds, antimicrobial activity and bioaccessibility studies with wild edible mushrooms. Food Science and Technology. 2015a;**63**:799-806

[13] Venturella G, Eristanna P, Filippo S, Maria LG. Notes on a new productive strain of king oyster mushroom, *Pleurotus eryngii* (higher Basidiomycetes), a prized Italian culinary medicinal mushroom. International Journal of Medicinal Mushrooms. 2015;**17**(2): 199-206

[14] Thatoi H, Sameer KS. Diversity, nutritional composition and medicinal potential of Indian mushrooms. African Journal of Biotechnology. 2014;**13**(4): 523-545

[15] Lange L. The importance of fungi and mycology for addressing major global challenges. IMAFungus. 2014; **5**(2):463-471

[16] Chaturvedi VK, Agarwal S, Gupta KK, Ramteke PW, Singh MP. Medicinal mushroom: Boon for therapeutic applications. 3 Biotech. 2018;**8**(8):334

[17] Lindequist U, Timo HJ, Niedermeyer Y, Julich W-D. The

pharmacological potential of mushroom. Evidence-based Complementary and Alternative Medicine. 2005;**2**(3):285-299

[18] El-Batal AI, El-Kenawy NM, Yassin AS, Amin MA. Laccase production by *Pleurotus ostreatus* and its application in synthesis of gold nanoparticles. Biotechnology Reports. 2015;**5**:31-39

[19] Zhang JJ, Li Y, Zhou T, et al. Bioactivities and Health Benefits of Mushrooms Mainly from China. Molecules. 2016;**21**(7):938

[20] Gadgil PD. Fungi on trees and shrubs in New Zealand. In: Fungi of New Zealand, Fungal Diversity Research Series 16. Vol. 4. Hong Kong: Fungal Diversity Press; 2005. pp. 437-458

[21] Maia TM, Lopes ST, Almeida JMG, Rosa LH, Sampaio JP, Goncalves P, et al. Evolution of mating systems in basidiomycetes and the genetic architecture underlying mating-type determination in the yeast *Leucosporidium scottii*. Genetics. 2015; **201**:75-89

[22] Mothana RAA, Awadh NAA, Jansen R, Lindequist U. Antiviral lanostanoid triterpenes from the fungus *Ganoderma freifferi*. International Journal of Medicicinal Mushroom. 2003; **74**:177-180

[23] Le XT, Le QHN, Pham ND, Duong VH, Dentinger BTM, Moncalvo J-M. *Tomophagus cattienensis* sp. nov., a new Ganodermataceae species from Vietnam: Evidence from morphology and ITS DNA barcodes. Mycological Progress. 2012;**11**:775-780

[24] Florian H, Zakaria C-A, Tim L, Jose GM-V, Helge BB, Meike P. Distinguishing commercially grown *Ganoderma lucidum* from *Ganoderma lingzhi* from Europe and East Asia on the basis of morphology, molecular phylogeny, and triterpenic acid profiles. Phytochemistry. 2016;**127**:29-37

[25] Liyanage ADS. Rubber. In: Hillocks RJ, Walter JM, editors. Soil Borne Diseases of Tropical Crops. Wallingford, UK: CAB International; 1997. pp. 331-347

[26] Oghenekaro AO, Miettinen O, Omorusi VI, Evueh GA, Farid MA, Gazis R, et al. Molecular phylogeny of *Rigidoporus microporus* isolates associated with white rot disease of rubber trees (*Hevea brasiliensis*). Fungal Biology. 2014;**18**:495-506

[27] Zhang M, Huang J, Xie X, Holman CD. Dietary intakes of mushrooms and green tea combine to reduce the risk of breast cancer in Chinese women. International Journal of Cancer. 2009;**124**(6): 1404-1408

[28] Chen SO, Phung SRS, Hur G, Ye JJ, Kwok SL, Shrode GE, et al. Anti-aromatase activity of phytochemicals in white button mushrooms (*Agaricus bisporus*). Cancer Research. 2006; **66**(24):1026-1034

[29] Deng G, Lin H, Seidman A. A phase I/II trial of polysaccharide extracts from *Grifola frondosa* (Maitake mushroom) in breast cancer patients: Immunological effects. Journal of Cancer Research and Clinical Oncology. 2009;**135**(9): 1215-1221

[30] Masuda Y, Murata Y, Hayashi M, Nanba H. Inhibitory effect of MD-fraction on tumor metastasis: Involvement of NK cell activation and suppression of intercellular adhesion molecule (ICAM)-1 expression in lung vascular endothelial cells. Biological and Pharmaceutical Bulletin. 2008;**31**(6): 1104-1124

[31] Regulo CLH, Michele LL, Anne-Marie F, Marie FO, Nathalie F,

Catherine RR, et al. Potential of European wild strains of *Agaricus subrufescens* for productivity and quality on wheat straw based compost. World Journal of Microbiology and Biotechnology. 2013;**29**(7):1243-1253

[32] Akinyele BJ, Ogidi CO. Towards potential utilization of wild and edible medicinal macrofungi indigenous to Nigeria as a source of anticancer agents. In: 7th Annual Submit on Microbiology: Education, Research and Development. San Antonio, Texas, USA; 2018

[33] Yeh JY, Hsieh LH, Wu KT, Tsai CF. Antioxidant properties and antioxidant compounds of various extracts from the edible basidiomycete *Grifola Frondosa* (Maitake). Molecules. 2011;**16**:3197-3211

[34] Kirk PM, Cannon PF, Minter DW, Stalpers JA. Dictionary of the Fungi. 10th ed. Wallingford, UK: CAB International; 2008. pp. 365-368

[35] Bisen PS, Baghel RK, Sanodiya BS, Thakur GS, Prasad GBKS. *Lentinus edodes*: A macrofungus with pharmacological activities. Current Medicinal Chemistry. 2010;**17**: 2419-2430

[36] Pegler DN. The genus *Lentinula* (*Tricholomataceae* tribe Collybieae). Sydowia. 1983;**36**:227-239

[37] Krishnamoorthy AS, Bala V. A comprehensive review of tropical milky white mushroom (*Calocybe indica* P and C). Mycobiology. 2015;**43**(3):184-194

[38] Stamets P. Growth parameters for gourmet and medicinal mushroom species. In: Growing Gourmet and Medicinal Mushrooms. 3rd ed. Berkeley, California, USA: Ten Speed Press; 2000. pp. 308-315

[39] Philips N, Roger F. Mushrooms. 6th ed. London, United Kingdom: Macmillan Publishers; 2006. 266p

[40] Stamets P. The role of mushrooms in nature. In: Growing Gourmet and Medicinal Mushrooms. 3rd ed. Berkeley, California, USA: Ten Speed Press; 2005. pp. 10-11

[41] Overholts LO. Geographical distribution of some American Polyporaceae. Mycologia. 1939;**13**(6): 629-652

[42] Rathod MM. Taxonomic studies on the daedaloid and hexagonoid polypores form the forest of Western Maharasta. Recent Research in Science and Technology. 2011;**3**(5):50-56

[43] Kirk PM. Species fungorum. In: Species 2000 and Integrated Taxonomic Information System (ITIS), Catalogue of Life. version 23rd. Leiden, The Netherlands: Naturalis; 2016. pp. 107-111

[44] Bhattacharjee B, Roy A, Majumder AL. Carboxymethylcellulase from *Lenzites saepiaria*, a brown-rotter. International Journal of Biochemistry and Molecular Biology. 1993;**30**(6): 1143-1152

[45] Baldrian P. Purification and characterization of laccase from the white-rot fungus; *Daedalea quercina* and decolorization of synthetic dyes by the enzyme. Applied Microbiology and Biotechnology. 2004; **63**(5):560-563

[46] Gilbertson RL. Wood-rotting fungi of North America. Mycologia. 1980; **72**(1):1-49

[47] Liu K, Wang JL, Gong WZ, Xiao X, Wang Q. Antioxidant activities *in vitro* of ethanol extract and fractions from mushroom, *Lenzites betulina*. Journal of Food Biochemistry. 2012;**37**(6): 687-693

[48] Cheung PCK. The nutritional and health benefits of mushrooms. Nutrition Bulletin. 2010;**35**:292-299

[49] Barros L, Cruz T, Baptista P, Estevinho LM, Ferreira ICFR. Wild and commercial mushrooms as source of nutrients and nutraceuticals. Food and Chemical Toxicology. 2008;**46**: 2742-2747

[50] Lallawmsanga, Passari AK, Mishra VK, Leo VV, Singh BP, Meyyappan GV, et al. Antimicrobial potential, identification and phylogenetic affiliation of wild mushrooms from two sub-tropical semi-evergreen Indian forest ecosystems. PLoS One. 2016;**11**(11): e0166368

[51] Kim M-Y, Chung I-M, Lee S-J, et al. Comparison of free amino acid, carbohydrates concentrations in Korean edible and medicinal mushrooms. Food Chemistry. 2009;**113**: 386-393

[52] Ogidi CO, Oyetayo VO, Akinyele BJ, De Carvalho CA, Kasuya MCM. Food value and safety status of raw (unfermented) and fermented higher basidiomycetes, *Lenzites quercina* (L) P. Karsten. Preventive Nutrition and Food Science. 2018;**23**(3):228-234

[53] Veera T, Jari M, Mikko K, Kauko S. Modelling the yields of marketed mushrooms in *Picea abies* stands in eastern Finland. Forest Ecology and Management. 2016;**362**:79-88

[54] Heleno SA, Ferreira RC, Antonio AL, Queiroz MRP, Barros L, Ferreira ICFR. Nutritional value, bioactive compounds and antioxidant properties of three edible mushrooms from Poland. Food Bioscience. 2015b;**11**: 48-55

[55] Badalyan SM. Potential of mushroom bioactive molecules to develop healthcare biotech products. In: Proceedings of the 8th International Conference on Mushroom Biology and Mushroom Products (ICMBMP8). New Dehli, India; 2014

[56] Enshasy H, Elsayed EA, Aziz R, Wadaan MA. Mushrooms and truffles: Historical biofactories for complementary medicine in Africa and in the Middle East. Evidence-based Complementary and Alternative Medicine. 2013;**2013**:1-10

[57] Rathore H, Prasad S, Sharma S. Mushroom nutraceuticals for improved nutrition and better human health: A review. Pharma Nutrition. 2017;**5**:35-46

[58] Cör D, Knez Ž, Knez Hrnčič M. Antitumour, Antimicrobial, Antioxidant and Antiacetylcholinesterase Effect of Ganoderma lucidum Terpenoids and Polysaccharides: A Review. Molecules. 2018;**23**(3):649

[59] Zhu F, Bin D, Zhaoxiang B, Xu B. Beta-glucans from edible and medicinal mushrooms: Characteristics, physicochemical and biological activities. Journal of Food Composition and Analysis. 2015;**41**:65-173

[60] Vetvicka V, Jana V. Immune enhancing effects of Maitake (*Grifola frondosa*) and shiitake (*Lentinula edodes*) extracts. Annals of Translational Medicine. 2014;**2**(2):14-16

[61] Kodama N, Komuta K, Akanda H. Effect of maitake (*Grifola frondosa*) D-fraction on the activation of NK cells in cancer patient. Journal of Medicinal Food. 2003;**6**:371-377

[62] Mothana RAA, Jansen R, Julich W-D, Lindequist U. Ganomycin a and B, new antimicrobial farnesyl hydroquinones from the Basidiomycete *Ganoderma pfeifferi*. Journal of Natural Products. 2000;**63**:416-418

[63] Oyetayo VO. Mushroom indigenous to Nigeria as potential source of myconutraceuticals. Biotechnology and Pharmarcy. 2008;**2**(4):471-477

[64] Yamasaki A, Shoda M, Iijima H, et al. A protein bound polysaccharide,

psk, enhances tumor suppression induced by docetaxel in a gastric cancer xenograft model. Anticancer Research. 2009;**29**(3):843-850

[65] Mursito B, Jenie UA, Mubarika S, Kardono KAB. Isolation of β-(1, 3) glucan, compound from the water extract of Indonesian Janur Tanduk [*Termitomynces eurirrhizus* (BSK)]. Journal of Biological Sciences. 2010;**13**: 187-195

[66] Goss PE, Strasser-Weipp K, Lee-Bychkovsky BL, Fan L, et al. Challenges to effective cancer control in China, India and Russia. The Lancet Oncology Commission. 2014;**15**:489-538

[67] Demain AL, Vaishnav P. Natural products for cancer chemotherapy. Microbial Biotechnology. 2011;**4**(6): 687-699

[68] Zhao YY. Traditional uses, phytochemistry, pharmacology, pharmacokinetics and quality control of *Polyporus umbellatus* (Pers.) fries: A review. Journal of Ethnopharmacology. 2013;**149**:35-48

[69] Jiang J, Sliva D. Novel medicinal mushroom blend suppresses growth and invasiveness of human breast cancer cells. International Journal of Oncology. 2010;**37**:1529-1536

[70] Ajith KA, Kainoor KJ. Indian medical mushroom as a source of antioxidant and anti-tumor agents. Journal of Clinical Biochemistry and Nutrition. 2007; **40**(3):157-162

[71] Jedinak AJ, Sliva D. *Pleurotus ostreatus* inhibits proliferation of human breast and colon cancer cells through p53-dependent as well as p53-independent pathway. International Journal of Oncology. 2008;**33**:1307-1313

[72] Patel S, Goyal A. Recent developments in mushrooms as anti-cancer therapeutics. 3. Biotech. 2012;**2**:1-15

[73] Upadhyay A, Indu U, Anup KJ, Kumar V. Combating pathogenic microorganisms using plant-derived antimicrobials: A mini review of the mechanistic basis. BioMed Research International. 2014;**2014**:1-18

[74] Mishra VK, Passari AK, Leo VV, Singh BP. Molecular diversity and detection of endophytic fungi based on their antimicrobial biosynthetic genes. In: Singh BP, Gupta VK, editors. Molecular Markers in Mycology, Fungal Biology. Switzerland: Springer International Publisher; 2016. pp. 1-35

[75] Ameri A, Vaidya JG, Deoku SS. *In vitro* evaluation of anti-staphylococcal activity of *Ganoderma lucidum*, *Ganoderma praelongum* and *Ganoderma resinaceum* from Pune, India. African Journal of Microbiology Research. 2011; **5**(3):328-333

[76] Abubakar Z, Ogidi CO, Oyetayo VO. Assessment of antistaphylococcal activity of ethanolic extract of *Lenzites quercina* (L) P. Karsten against clinical *Staphylococcus* species. Clinical Phytoscience. 2016; **2**(8):1-7

[77] Bender S, Dumitrache CN, Backhaus J, Christie G, Lonergan GT. A case for caution in assessing the antibiotic activity of culinary medicinal shiitake mushroom (*Lentinus edodes* (BSK) sings). International Journal of Medicinal Mushroom. 2003;**5**:31-35

[78] Zjawiony J. Biologically active compounds from Aphyllophorales (polypore) Fungi. Journal of Natural Products. 2004;**67**:300-310

[79] El-Fakharany EM, Haroun BM, Ng TB, Redwan ER. Oyster mushroom laccase inhibits hepatitis C virus entry into peripheral blood cells and

hepatoma cells. Protein and Peptide Letters. 2010;**17**:1031-1039

[80] Wang H, Ng TB. Isolation of a novel ubiquitin-like protein from *Pleurotus ostreatus* mushroom with anti-human immune deficiency virus, translation-inhibitory and Ribonuclease activities. Biochemical Biophysiology Research Community. 2000;**276**: 587-593

[81] Karacsonyi S, Kuniak L. Polysaccharides of *Pleurotus ostreatus*: Isolation and structure of pleuran, an alkali-insoluble beta-D-glucan. Carbohydrate Polymers. 1994;**24**: 107-111

[82] Deepalakshmi K, Mirunalini S. *Pleurotus ostreatus*: An oyster mushroom with nutritional and medicinal properties. Journal of Biochemical Technology. 2014;**5**(2): 718-726

[83] Karaman M, Jovin E, Malbasa R, Matavuly M, Popovie M. Medicinal and edible lignicolous fungi as natural source of antioxidative and antibacterial agents. Phytotheraphy Research. 2010; **24**:1473-1481

[84] Mirunalini S, Arulmozhi V, Deepalakshmi K, Krishnaveni M. Intracellular biosynthesis and antibacterial activity of silver nanoparticles using edible mushrooms. Notulae Scientia Biologicae. 2012;**4**(4): 55-61

[85] Sen S, Chakraborty R, Sridhar C, Reddy YSR, De B. Free radicals, antioxidants, diseases and phytomedicines: Current status and future prospect. International Journal of Pharmaceutical Sciences Review and Research. 2010;**3**(1):91-100

[86] Halliwell B, Gutteridge J. Free Radicals in Biology and Medicine. 4th ed. Oxford, UK: Oxford University Press; 2007. pp. 58-59

[87] Valko M, Leibfritz D, Moncol J, Cronin MT, Mazur M, Telser J. Free radicals and antioxidants in normal physiological functions and human diseases. International Journal of Biochemistry and Cell Biology. 2007;**39**: 44-84

[88] Ekin S, Uzun Y, Kenan D, Mahire B, Hatice K. Chemical composition and antioxidant activity of two wild edible mushrooms from Turkey. International Journal of Medicinal Mushrooms. 2015; **17**(12):1179-1188

[89] Ferreira ICFR, Barros L, Abreu RMV. Antioxidants in wild mushrooms. Current Medicinal Chemistry. 2009;**16**:1543-1560

[90] Xu L, Wang Q, Guiqiang W, Wub JY. Contents and antioxidant activities of polysaccharides in 14 wild mushroom species from the forest of northeastern China. International Journal of Medicinal Mushrooms. 2015; **17**(12):1161-1170

[91] Cai M, Lin Y, Luo Y, Liang H, Sun P. Extraction, antimicrobial, and antioxidant activities of crude polysaccharides from the wood ear medicinal mushroom *Auricularia auricula-judae* (higher Basidiomycetes). International Journal of Medicinal Mushrooms. 2015;**17**(6):591-600

[92] Kalaras MD, Richie JP, Calcagnotto A, Beelman RB. Mushrooms: A rich source of the antioxidants ergothioneine and glutathione. Food Chemistry. 2017;**33**: 429-433

[93] Manohar V, Talpur NA, Echard BW, Lieberman S, Preuss HG. Effects of a water-soluble extract of maitake mushroom on circulating glucose/ insulin concentrations in KK mice. Diabetes Obes Metab. 2002;**4**(1):43-48

[94] Wu Y-Y, Xiao E, Graves DT. *Diabetes mellitus* related bone

metabolism and periodontal disease. International Journal of Oral Science. 2015;7:63-72

[95] Hsu T-H, Lee C-H, Lin FY, Wasser SP, Lo H-C. The fruiting bodies, submerged culture biomass, and acidic polysaccharide glucuronoxylomannan of yellow brain mushroom *Tremella mesenterica* modulate the immunity of peripheral blood leukocytes and splenocytes in rats with impaired glucose tolerance. Journal of Traditional and Complementary Medicine. 2014; **4**(1):56-63

[96] Ogbole OO, Nkumah AO, Linus AU, Falade MO. Molecular identification, *in vivo* and *in vitro* activities of *Calvatia gigantea* (macrofungus) as an antidiabetic agent. Mycology: An International Journal on Fungal Biology. 2019;**31;10**(3):166-173

[97] Ogidi CO. Molecular identification and assessment of some nutraceutical potentials of a wild macrofungus; *Lenzites quercina* [Ph.D thesis]. Akure, Nigeria: Department of Microbiology, The Federal University of Technology; 2017

[98] Ogidi CO, Oyetayo VO, Akinyele BJ, Ogbole OO, Adeniji AJ, Oluremi BB. Molecular identity and cytotoxicity of extracts obtained from macrofungus; *Lenzites quercina* against cancer cell lines. Journal of Biotechnology, Computational Biology and Bionanotechnology: BioTechnologia. 2017;**98**(1):25-32

[99] Osemwegie OO, Okhuoya AJ, Dania AT. Ethnomycological conspectus of west African mushrooms: An awareness document. Advances in Microbiology. 2014;**4**:39-54

[100] Oyetayo VO. Medicinal uses of mushrooms in Nigeria: Towards full and sustainable exploitation. African Journal of Traditional, Complementary, and Alternative Medicines. 2011;**8**(3): 267-274